S. Hrg. 113–687

COMMUNITY SOLUTIONS TO BREAKING THE CYCLE OF HEROIN AND OPIOID ADDICTION

HEARING

BEFORE THE

COMMITTEE ON THE JUDICIARY
UNITED STATES SENATE

ONE HUNDRED THIRTEENTH CONGRESS

FIRST SESSION

MONDAY, MARCH 17, 2014

RUTLAND, VERMONT

Serial No. J–113–53

Printed for the use of the Committee on the Judiciary

U.S. GOVERNMENT PUBLISHING OFFICE

95–645 PDF   WASHINGTON : 2015

For sale by the Superintendent of Documents, U.S. Government Publishing Office
Internet: bookstore.gpo.gov Phone: toll free (866) 512–1800; DC area (202) 512–1800
Fax: (202) 512–2104 Mail: Stop IDCC, Washington, DC 20402–0001

CONTENTS

STATEMENTS OF COMMITTEE MEMBERS

WITNESSES

QUESTIONS

ANSWERS

SUBMISSIONS FOR THE RECORD

COMMUNITY SOLUTIONS TO BREAKING THE CYCLE OF HEROIN AND OPIOID ADDICTION

MONDAY, MARCH 17, 2014

U.S. SENATE,
COMMITTEE ON THE JUDICIARY,
Washington, DC.

The Committee met, pursuant to notice, at 1:07 p.m., in the Franklin Conference Center at the Howe Center, 1 Scale Avenue, Rutland, Vermont, Hon. Patrick J. Leahy, Chairman of the Committee, presiding.

Present: Senator Leahy.

Also present: Representative Welch.

OPENING STATEMENT OF HON. PATRICK J. LEAHY, A U.S. SENATOR FROM THE STATE OF VERMONT

Chairman LEAHY. If we can all come to order. I want to thank everybody for being here, including Congressman Welch, because this is a bicameral matter. I must point out that Congressman Welch has a much brighter green tie on than I do.

First off, I will wish all of you a Happy St. Patrick's Day, and thank you for coming out for this.

We are having this hearing—and I know so many of you in this room and I have worked with so many of you here in Rutland—to talk about opioid addiction and heroin and how communities such as Rutland can successfully come together to solve this complex problem.

It is a complex challenge. It goes into neighborhoods, it goes into communities of all kinds and sizes, in urban and rural areas alike throughout the country. And Vermont has not been spared. We have seen that the demand for treatment between the year 2012 for addiction in Vermont rose by more than 770 percent, and Dr. Chen can speak about this in greater detail. But that is consistent with what we are seeing with opioids around the country, including heroin. We also hear the stories of the young people whose lives have either been ruined or ended because of this.

Now, Vermont is way ahead of the country in many ways. We have openly identified the problem. We are trying to find ways to not just help addicts get clean, but to stop this. We have heard many times, but it bears repeating, and I would say this as somebody who spent eight years as a State's attorney: You cannot arrest your way out of this problem. It is not just a law enforcement problem even though we have among the finest law enforcement people in the country. You cannot just put it on the backs of law enforcement. You have to have prevention, education, and treatment to go along with law enforcement.

(1)

We have many eyes now on Vermont. Governor Shumlin has spoken forcefully about the heroin crisis. It is significant that he did something no other Governor in the country would do. He dedicated his State of the State message to this problem this year.

The Chief Justice of Vermont, Paul Reiber, has added his voice. He noted, "This challenge is complex and cannot only be met with the blunt tool of criminalization."

This addiction is an issue of great importance to me, both as a lifelong Vermonter but also as someone who cares deeply about making sure we have a legal, lasting solution. And I want to applaud Rutland. Rutland has been in the forefront of seeking solutions and working hard to do it. This city is one I have known from my childhood days on, and it is a city that deserves enormous admiration for what it does. But we have to get ahead of addiction. We cannot let it corrode our lives and our communities.

Now, I look at problems in our criminal justice system at the federal level. What I see is that when we look for creative solutions, many times the solutions we find at the federal level are actually being done at the local level. And if we look at what has been tried in a community like this, it sometimes sets the model for what we should do nationally. If it works in the State system, we ought to adopt it at the federal system. And Vermonters do not shy from a challenge, and they do not hesitate to tell you what is on their mind. And so we have got some innovative programs.

Chief Baker is working collaboratively with Mayor Louras and residents—and I saw the mayor at lunch right around the corner—and community developers, housing advocates, and prevention specialists. A community response known as Project VISION shows how people can join together to combat drugs. The Project VISION'S Chairman, Joe Kraus, summed it up this way: "We have two choices here. We can curse the darkness, or we can light a candle, to quote an old saying."

Well, Rutland is just one example of how communities around Vermont are working together to confront this crisis. It is not unique just to the large cities. As Sheriff Roger Marcoux notes in his written testimony, which will be part of the record, roughly half of Vermont's overdoses since 2011 have occurred in rural settings. [The prepared statement of Sheriff Marcoux appears as a submission for the record.]

Chairman LEAHY. I live on a dirt road in Vermont in a town of 1,500 people. My nearest neighbor is a half a mile away. I do not think that we face any less of a problem there than you do in our largest cities.

We have to be in it together. This is the fourth time I have brought the Judiciary Committee here to Vermont, and we have talked about the three-tiered approach: prevention, treatment, and enforcement. But Vermont has shown that more success is possible when prevention and treatment and law enforcement are not each one in a little section by themselves. And I know from my own years in law enforcement as State's attorney in Chittenden County how important these efforts are.

I have never seen in my lifetime in this State a law enforcement community more fully committed to prevention and treatment efforts as we have right now. And I think we Vermonters ought to be proud of that because law enforcement would rather not arrest and prosecute the same offenders over and over again when what you have is a treatable addiction. And treating the addiction can be the better and less costly approach. It also results in a lot fewer cases lying on detectives' and prosecutors' desks.

One of the programs I am working on in Washington is the *Second Chance Act*. We have introduced it for reauthorization. It is going to be coming before the Senate Judiciary Committee very soon. It supports initiatives like the Vermont Court Diversion Program so that people with minor charges can keep their records clean if they successfully complete a program. Otherwise, how are these people ever going to be hired? How are they ever going to get a job?

We have seen innovative diversion models that have emerged in response to community needs. We saw in Windsor County the Sparrow Project, Rapid Intervention efforts in Chittenden County. Those are just a few examples. But we also have witnesses who are going to talk about how we break the cycle of addiction in our communities. Vermont's superb U.S. Attorney, Tris Coffin, has taken his message of prevention into Vermont's schools, and, Tris, I know you have also gone with the father of a University of Vermont student, who died of a heroin overdose. And I get letters and I get calls from people when you have both been there to talk to them, so thank you for doing that.

Chief Baker is facilitating a community-based response. He boils it down to a very simple Vermont message: "Not on our streets, not in our town." That sort of says it all, Chief.

Chief BAKER. Thank you, Senator.

Chairman LEAHY. Dr. Chen, with his years of experience as an emergency room physician, is now working with the Governor to take the prevention message to our communities and to our schools.

Mary Alice McKenzie, whom I have known all her life, and her parents before that, is working through the Boys & Girls Clubs to respond to the needs of our kids. And I think you have found these kids want a positive and healthy and supportive alternative to addiction.

And the Vermont State Police under the direction of Colonel L'Esperance, in partnership with the Vermont Department of Health, are using a promising drug, naloxone, which can immediately reverse the effects of a heroin overdose. The colonel met with me in my office in Montpelier here a few weeks ago to show me that.

So I really want to hear from all of you, but before I do, I am going to turn to Congressman Welch. One of the lucky things in Vermont, we all know each other and we can work together. Peter Welch had a distinguished career in the State legislature before he went to the House. He is well respected on both sides of the aisle, and I think it is safe to say we both found the same thing, that this is not a Republican or a Democratic issue. It is a human issue. And for us in this room, it is a Vermont issue. Peter.

OPENING STATEMENT OF HON. PETER WELCH, A REPRESENTATIVE IN CONGRESS FROM THE STATE OF VERMONT

Representative WELCH. Patrick, thank you.

I want to thank Patrick, because I know everybody else does, for bringing the Judiciary Committee here. And with your eight years—was it eight years that you were the Chittenden County State's attorney?

Chairman LEAHY. Yes.

Representative WELCH. Oftentimes you speak about that as a job above all others where you were dealing with real people and real lives, and that experience, obviously, is what a lot of our panelists share and a lot of Vermonters here share. And now you happen to be the most senior member of the U.S. Senate and in a position to really help us help the people who are trying to help Rutland. So we are all very grateful to you, Patrick, for convening this hearing here today. I just want to give him a round of applause.

[Applause.]

Representative WELCH. And I cannot add to what Patrick said, but, you know, as a Vermonter—we are all Vermonters, and the kind of thing that binds us together is we have this almost indiscriminate pride about our sense of place and sense of community, that it is small, that we care about our neighbors. And there was a lot of alarm, to some extent, when the Governor spoke in his whole address about this challenge. And some folks were a bit nervous that we were giving publicity to a "bad problem."

But you know what? What we know is that when communities face their problems, it is the first step in solving their problems. And it was interesting to me in Congress, I had colleagues from all over the country who saw the publicity, and they came up to me, and they said, "Peter, how do you guys get the nerve to do this? Because this is a problem we are facing, but we are not dealing with it."

And if we are going to maintain what it is we find so important to each of us, a sense of community, it means we have got to step up and not look to the courts as the sole solution or to our law enforcement as the sole solution, but where we acknowledge every one of us really has a role to play.

One of the things that has been so great for me in watching this is that it has given parents some space to come out of the shadows and talk to their other parents about, "Is this a problem for you?" And they can get the support they need to try to cope.

So, Patrick, this hearing, I think all of us are really grateful to you, and I want to echo your remarks, too, that the real heroes here are the moms and the dads and the citizens of Rutland and of the State of Vermont who are stepping up to work together to try to do everything we can to mitigate and minimize this issue. Thank you.

Chairman LEAHY. Thank you very much.

[Applause.]

Chairman LEAHY. I cannot applaud Rutland enough, because we had a similar hearing a few years ago when Senator Arlen Specter and I were here, and that shaped a number of federal programs for the better because of what we heard from you.

Our first witness is Tristram Coffin, the U.S. Attorney for the District of Vermont. He grew up in South Burlington, graduated from Columbia Law School, clerked for Federal District Court Judge Albert Coffrin. In the early 1990s, he helped make the Senate Judiciary Committee better by serving on that staff in Washington.

He came back here, was for 12 years Assistant U.S. Attorney, went back into private practice after specializing in international drug-smuggling cases, and worked with the Canadian law enforcement. But the President asked him to step out of private practice, and he became the 36th U.S. Attorney for the District of Vermont in 2009.

Before we begin, Tris, I want to applaud you for the fact that I hear from State police, local police, county police in the State how much you and your office have worked with them.

STATEMENT OF HON. TRISTRAM COFFIN, U.S. ATTORNEY, DISTRICT OF VERMONT, DEPARTMENT OF JUSTICE, BURLINGTON, VERMONT

Mr. COFFIN. Thank you, Senator. Thank you very much. It is such an honor to be here today with our partners in all these activities, and I want to thank you, Senator, for bringing the Senate Judiciary Committee to Vermont and for inviting me to share with you my views about the need for a broader community reaction to heroin and other opiate trafficking, use, and addiction. I and the Department of Justice appreciate your leadership on these issues for so many years and your dedication to improving the lives of Vermonters.

First let me say that Rutland is a terrific small city. It has a strong and proud community and a great tradition. But it is a community like many others throughout New England and the United States that is going through a difficult time right now.

Many communities are having to face up to the many significant challenges that are presented by opioid trafficking and addiction. Rutland is addressing these problems in a forthright, aggressive, and creative fashion. I commend Chief Baker and the rest of the Rutland community for doing that.

The heroin, opiate, and opioid problem in Vermont is not new. It has been building for some time. Under your leadership, Senator Leahy, this Judiciary Committee has held three field hearings in Vermont on the issue of drugs in recent years, including opiates. As the problem of opioid addiction began to emerge, you invited Attorney General Holder here for the Opiate Prescription Medication and Heroin Summit we held in Montpelier in September 2010. You stated back then that the problem that was existing of rampant addiction to opioid prescription medications would soon lead to substantial heroin trafficking and addiction in Vermont, and, unfortunately, that indeed has happened.

On March 10, 2014, Attorney General Holder in a public video message called the rise in overdose deaths from heroin and other prescription painkillers "an urgent public health crisis." I could not agree more.

The numbers and statistics are stark. Between 2006 and 2010, heroin overdose deaths decreased nationally by 45 percent. Heroin treatment numbers in Vermont are up over 250 percent since 2000 and over 40 percent in the past year. Our office's prosecution of heroin traffickers is up, with indictments more than doubling last year and totaling more than four times what they were just a few years ago.

But to me, one of the starkest statistics is the increase in fatal heroin overdoses we have here in Vermont. Last year's total—a record 21—was more than twice the number of the year before, which was also a record. And that is five times the number of what we had just a few years ago.

These are obviously extremely concerning numbers. I want to echo the Attorney General and urge first responders to carry the drug known as naloxone. When administered quickly and effectively, naloxone immediately restores breathing to a victim in the throes of a heroin or opioid overdose. I applaud the Vermont State Police and the Vermont Department of Health for moving forward on this issue.

When you deal with the families of overdose victims, I can tell you that every one of these numbers has a face and a name and loved ones left behind in pain that does not go away.

The Justice Department, along with our partners in the Vermont State Police and Rutland Police Department, has been aggressive about prosecuting traffickers who seek to profit out of selling this misery, and we will continue to do so. But what this hearing is about is how important it is for the community to respond as a whole to this problem. We will remain active and vigilant on the law enforcement side, but it is not enough. This problem requires a broad community response, and I am thrilled that under the leadership of Chief Baker and others, Rutland is engaged in making this response, and similar broad community responses to this problem are happening throughout other parts of Vermont as well.

Attorney General Holder has been very clear with me and my fellow U.S. Attorneys that we need to be smarter on crime, not just tougher. We are not giving the community what it deserves if we offer up only an expensive solution—unlimited incarceration—if it does not address the root causes of the problem.

When we look at the problem of heroin and opioid use, law enforcement alone is not sufficient to address the problem. Community responses emphasizing prevention and treatment are essential complements to work in conjunction with law enforcement to make the community a safer and more drug-free place.

Over the last three years, I have been fortunate to be involved in one such prevention program. On March 23, 2009, Skip Gates lost his treasured son, Will, to a heroin overdose. Will was an outstanding young man. He was in his third year at the University of Vermont studying molecular genetics, a standout Alpine ski racer, an incredible young man. We met Skip through the investigation of the heroin trafficker who sold Will the heroin that led to his death. Skip was searching for some way to turn this tragedy into something positive. Working with our office's outstanding crime victim advocate, Aimee Stearns, who I think is here today, and a great young filmmaker named Derek Hallquist, who is here, Skip, who is also present, had the courage to share his personal experience of this tragedy in the short film "The Opiate Effect." We have sent the film to all the high schools in Vermont for free two years running. Also with the help from our office, Jim Lean, our law enforcement coordinator, we have spent the last three years traveling throughout Vermont playing the movie and talking to high school kids and their parents about the dangers of opioid use. Skip is an eloquent speaker, and the film is powerful. I think a lot of the power of the movie comes from its informational approach. Young people see firsthand the impact heroin has had on Skip and on his family. They hear from recovering addicts straight talk about what life as a heroin addict is like. The film does not really try to moralize; rather, it lays out the real facts on what life as an opioid addict is like so people can make clear choices. In this way, the film moves the conversation beyond "Just Say No."

The importance of this, of course, is to try to stop people from entering the opioid addiction and criminal justice pipeline, because once that happens, there are no good outcomes, only varying degrees of bad ones.

That is why the prospect of effective drug prevention is so important. We do a lot of work to reduce the supply of drugs coming into this State on the law enforcement side. But if we do not equally be as aggressive on reducing the demand side, our efforts will be of little avail.

We need better and more drug treatment to get people who are addicted to these substances off of them, and we need better and more comprehensive prevention approaches to reduce the number of people who fall into this trap. Law enforcement is not the only answer. We need these other efforts as well.

And to be successful, these prevention and treatment efforts must come from broad segments of the community, like those occurring here in Rutland and also in Burlington and many other communities in Vermont. We have to have realistic discussions of the issues communities face from opiate and other substance abuse and look to the ingenuity and creativity in these communities for newer and broader solutions.

And when we have these discussions, we need to understand that comprehensive approaches rather than piecemeal or solely law enforcement-oriented approaches are necessary to solve the problem, comprehensive solutions rooted in the particular community that make sense for their community and tailored to each community's unique situation and characteristics, solutions that draw upon the perspectives, skills, and insights of a variety of stakeholders, not just the police.

The other witnesses today, I know, will have much to add on this score, so I will close my remarks. But let me do so by thanking you, Senator Leahy, for coming here today and permitting me to speak on behalf of the Justice Department. And, moreover, thank you for your substantial dedication to this issue and your caring leadership on it for many years.

[The prepared statement of Mr. Coffin appears as a submission for the record.]

Chairman LEAHY. Thank you very much, and you and Skip should know that that film, which is powerful, is part of the permanent records of the Senate Judiciary Committee, and a lot of people have seen it.

Our next witness is Chief James Baker. Chief Baker served as head of the Vermont State Police for over 30 years before he retired in 2009. In 2012, he returned to public service and serves as Chief of the Rutland City Police. He has been recognized by everybody from the New England Narcotics Enforcement Association, Vermont Chiefs of Police Association, Vermont Sheriffs Association, Vermont Governor's Highway Safety Office, and the United States Attorney's Office. He is a graduate of Southern Vermont College, the FBI National Academy at Quantico, Virginia, and he is leading Rutland's community-based effort.

So, Chief, please go ahead.

STATEMENT OF JAMES W. BAKER, CHIEF, RUTLAND CITY POLICE DEPARTMENT, RUTLAND, VERMONT

Chief BAKER. Thank you, Senator.

AUDIENCE MEMBER. Could you stand up, please?

Chairman LEAHY. That is okay. I think with the microphones it is best he be right there. Just bring the microphone close.

Chief BAKER. Thank you. Senator, Representative Welch, on behalf of Mayor Louras, Mr. David Allaire, the president of the Board of Aldermen, elected officials of the city of Rutland, members of the Police Commission, the citizens of Rutland, and the men and women of the Rutland City Police Department, I welcome you to this great city.

We are proud of this great city, and we are honored you have taken the time to conduct a field hearing to hear about the good work being done here and the challenges of substance abuse and, in particular, opiate abuse.

I want to echo the comments of U.S. Attorney Tris Coffin. The city of Rutland is a terrific community with a strong and proud history. This hearing is being held in a building that represents Rutland's proud history. The building dates back to the 1800s when the Howe Scale Company was located here. After years of productive output, Howe Scale fell on hard times, and the company closed in the early 1980s, leaving this expansive manufacturing complex, with more than 330,000 square feet, vacant. What to do with this vast structure soon became the source of intense public debate and disagreement.

The debate about the future of the Howe Center has been captured and memorialized. It serves as a reminder of the challenges Rutland has faced. It serves as a reminder of the grit of this city. Just as Rutland created a new vision for the Howe Center, we are committed to remaking Rutland into one of the healthiest and safest cities in the United States. In fact, the Vision Statement of Project VISION is: "Healthiest, safest, and happiest community in America!" We have the people, the infrastructure and the will to get it done.

Not unlike other communities, the city of Rutland has faced the challenges of illegal drug activity before. In the early 1990s, as a young supervisor of a multi-agency drug task force, I worked out of Rutland and was involved in countless undercover drug operations that resulted in arrests, prosecutions, and convictions for drug distribution. The drugs of choice at the time were cocaine and marijuana. At that time, as a young investigator, I was convinced that the resources and efforts we applied had solved the drug problem. Fourteen years later, I became the director of the Vermont State Police, and Rutland City Police Chief, Tony Bossi, sought help from the State Police with a new and emerging drug problem. The call for help was based on a fatal shooting on Grove Street during a drug deal and reports of violence involving firearms. The city had reached the tipping point on drug activity and violence. After a significant commitment of resources, a drug sweep rounded up more than 40 defendants in an operation known as Operation Marble Valley. The cases had strong out-of-State influences marked with a serious presence of gun culture and the drugs involved were cocaine, crack cocaine, and heroin. At the press conference announcing the arrests, officials made the point that these arrests were meant to change the direction of the drug culture in Rutland. Around the same time under your leadership, Senator Leahy, the U.S. Senate Judiciary Committee held a field hearing in this very room. There was testimony about the need for prevention, treatment, and enforcement. The community rallied for a period of time. In January 2012, I arrived as the interim Chief of Police to find yet another emerging drug culture and challenge. This time, the drug was heroin. I found a police department that was demoralized and a community that had no trust in its police department. This dispirited atmosphere stemmed from the fact that there was an unrealistic expectation that the police department could and should singlehandedly resolve the issues of illegal drugs in the community.

As more pressure was applied to the police department to act, the more aggressive the law enforcement actions became. The measure of success was the number of arrests made and the amount of drugs seized. The trouble with those metrics was that history clearly showed that arrests alone were not going to change the environment because it does not take into account the underlying social issues relating to drugs. Not one of the underlying issues that are tied to addiction is under the control of the police, yet the solutions to the issue were laid at the doorstep of the police department. It became apparent that in order to effect change in our escalating drug crisis—a crisis from our experience that originates at its base from the initial addiction to prescription drugs—the situation was going to require all hands on deck.

As we began the conversation with our non-law enforcement partners, we worked to gather a coalition of local, State, county, and federal enforcement partners in an effort to change the culture and the environment on the street by employing laser-focused enforcement operations. The effort resulted in Operation Fedup and was coordinated by ATF and other partners, both federal, State, and local. The very first operation resulted in seizing nearly 8,000 bags of heroin and approximately $90,000 in cash. That investigation led to connections of drug distribution networks in New York City. The furtherance of the investigation under the guidance of U.S. Attorney Coffin, the DEA, and FBI revealed an organization that was responsible for bringing up to 10,000 bags of heroin into the Rutland area on a continual 10- to 14-day daily basis. It was hard to fathom the depth of the addiction in this area that would require that amount of heroin. We were all shocked. This was our first epiphany. We could no longer follow the methods deployed in the past if we were going to move the ball down the field. The demand for opiates was outstripping our ability to be effective.

The second epiphany came on September 26, 2012, at about 6 p.m. on Cleveland Ave in the city of Rutland, Vermont. It was on that day that we lost one of our bright and upcoming stars. Carly Ferro, age 17, was leaving her place of work and entering into her father's car to drive home when she was struck and killed. Carly was killed when a car operated by an individual who is alleged in court papers to have been huffing aerosols lost control of the car and struck her. The incident represented another critical point in Rutland's history where the grit and determination of her people was defined. This tragedy became a rallying point—a painful realization that what was happening in our city had to stop. The human costs were too high.

The non-traditional partners we had assembled became focused on creating metrics to measure where we were, and where we needed to go. We began meeting on a regular basis and began to follow a path and a model championed by Chief Mike Schirling of the Burlington Police Department known as Community Intervention Team. The vision was to join all resources together and create a multiplier force to affect the quality of life in Rutland. We brought to the table social services agencies, elected officials, police resources, the domestic violence advocacy community, drug court, corrections, prosecutors at the federal, State, and local level, economic development officials, housing coalition officials, the faith community, mediation services, neighborhood citizens, and many others.

In the early stages, the group talked and worked on strategies to create metrics using data to measure what success looked like. We worked on supporting and advocating for a methadone clinic. We worked on systems to better communicate across traditional and non-traditional partners. The energy was amazing.

The final epiphany came when Senator Leahy's staff located a grant opportunity from the United States Department of Justice Bureau of Justice Assistance. Our coalition refocused and developed a grant application that created the name Project VISION, known as Viable Initiatives & Solutions through Involvement of Neighborhoods). The grant created a blueprint using outcome-based modeling that we are following to execute our strategy.

We did not receive the grant. We think our good friends at BJA may have gotten this one wrong. But we did not give up.

Chairman LEAHY. They did get it wrong.

[Laughter.]

Chief BAKER. The grit and determination of Rutland shined once again, and we moved forward. We continued to execute our strategy, and we now have an operating structure in place. We have stayed faithful to the concept of utilizing research to validate our processes.

Project VISION serves as an umbrella group that coordinates the functions of three committees. Those committees are Crime and Safety; Substance Abuse, Prevention, and Treatment; and Neighborhoods and Housing. Each committee is working on unique goals to their individual committee with the understanding that they stay faithful to Project VISION's key values of collaboration for the greater good and renewed focus on the positive.

As a result of the collaboration of resources, the Rutland City Police Department is now host to a variety of non-traditional partners who operate on the guiding principle that the issues we face associated with substance abuse, mental health issues, and quality of life in our neighborhoods are interconnected. That interconnection requires an integrated response.

Today, housed in the Rutland City Police Department building, we have two social workers from the Rutland County Family and Children Center, a domestic violence advocate from the Rutland County Women's Network and Shelter, an Assistant Attorney General, an emergency crisis intervention specialist from Rutland County Mental Health, a Rutland County early intervention coordinator from the Rutland County State's Attorney's Office, a school resource officer, an animal control officer, a crime analyst, and—on a part-time basis—a City of Rutland building inspector. These resources are coordinated by Captain Scott Tucker, the newly named executive director of Project VISION and the commander of the newly formed Community Outreach Division in the Rutland City Police Department.

In the police department, we are embracing data and technology to identify where we apply these coordinated resources: never missing an opportunity to do a case review, create a system of better communications, and providing focused prosecution for those causing the most harm to our community. The effort coordinated daily is brought together on a bi-weekly basis when all committee members attend a mapping meeting. In the mapping meetings we look at the locations and individuals that are doing the most harm to our community. Based on that data, we develop integrated solutions to address each of those individual situations. As an example, in many cases the underlying issues of substance abuse and/or mental health issues have led to family violence or neighborhood unrest. By having all the resources at the table, we can develop strategies and a response that include more than a police response. Unlike in the past, police suppression is not our first or our only choice. We are working at root-cause issues.

It is important to note that we do still support and apply aggressive law enforcement to deal with those who choose not to meet our community norms and who do serious harm. As an example, the sources of heroin that make a conscious decision to come to Rutland to deal need to understand that their behavior is not going to be accepted or tolerated. That is why we work closely with the Vermont Drug Task Force and our federal partners to apply enforcement resources. We pay close attention to those who choose to do harm in the form of violence against women and children, not accepting that addiction is the cause.

To demonstrate the determination of this great city, I would ask anyone in the room who is associated in any way with Project VISION to please raise your hands.

Chairman LEAHY. That answers that question.

[Applause.]

Chairman LEAHY. I would note for the record, because this will be a part of the permanent record of the U.S. Senate, that at least half the hands in the room went up. And then they were applauded. I think that tells the story right there.

Go ahead, Chief.

Chief BAKER. Senator, these are the faces of determination in our community.

As I close, I want to thank all those partners who have worked to make our story worthy of telling in front of this Committee. There are too many to mention, but you know who you are.

Senator, I want to thank you, Representative Welch, I want to thank you. Senator Leahy, thank you for your unwavering support of the city of Rutland. It is appreciated by all of us who are working tirelessly to get this right.

Thank you.

[The prepared statement of Chief Baker follows:]

Chairman LEAHY. Well, thank you.

[Applause.]

Chairman LEAHY. Rutland is a city well worth helping. It is an integral and important part of Vermont, and we Vermonters treasure it.

Dr. Harry Chen was appointed Commissioner of the Vermont Department of Health by Governor Shumlin in January 2011. Before that, he spent 20 years as an emergency physician at Rutland Regional Medical Center and served as medical director from 1998 to 2004. I mention that because Dr. Chen knows this area very well. He had previously been on the faculty at GW University Medical Center, and now also teaches at the University of Vermont College of Medicine. He was a member of the Vermont House of Representatives. John Tracy in my office tells me how important it was to him that you were on the Health Care Committee and served as vice chair of that Committee.

Dr. Chen, I could go on about you all afternoon, but I will let you speak for yourself. Please go ahead, sir.

STATEMENT OF HARRY L. CHEN, M.D., COMMISSIONER OF HEALTH, BURLINGTON, VERMONT

Dr. CHEN. Thank you, Senator Leahy, and my sincere thanks for holding this hearing to highlight this extremely important issue.

Vermont brought the problem of addiction to heroin and other opioid drugs to national attention this year. You have heard about the stark numbers. More than 50 Vermonters die each year from opioid overdoses. Deaths from heroin have doubled between 2012 and 2013, and nearly 4,000 Vermonters are in treatment for opioid addiction; over half of them, tragically, are young adults. And even more are waiting for treatment.

Vermont's experience has become the talk of the Nation, and, alas, for good reason. If it can happen here, in a mostly rural State made up of close-knit communities, blessed with natural beauty, where health care is nearly universal, with residents recognized as being among the healthiest of Americans, it can happen anywhere. From my viewpoint, addiction must be recognized as a public health problem and treated as a chronic illness. Addiction results from bad decisions. Those bad decisions quickly move to a disease. The end result is a chronic medical condition with profound implications for the individual and society. That is why Vermont is taking a comprehensive public health approach to the problem of substance abuse and addiction that involves prevention, early identification and intervention, an array of treatment services, and recovery supports.

It is now well accepted that we cannot simply arrest our way out of the problem. A bill passed just last week by the Vermont Senate acknowledges that by diverting non-violent drug offenders from the criminal justice system, instead referring them to treatment as soon as possible.

And addiction is not someone else's problem. It is our problem. As a longtime former resident and physician in the Rutland area, I, along with virtually everybody in this room, can point to good kids from good families whose lives were taken over by the horrors of opiate addiction.

With the opening of the West Ridge Addiction Treatment & Recovery Center in November 2013, we marked a milestone in Rutland County and for our State. We now acknowledge that addiction is a chronic illness, like diabetes and heart disease, requiring a similar approach to prevention and treatment. We believe we are on the right path. Let me describe our path in a little more detail.

The Vermont Department of Health has prevention consultants in our 12 district offices, including Rutland. Their role as local experts is to educate community members, help organize prevention efforts, and support coalitions with technical assistance to help implement proven prevention strategies. We are fortunate to have a series of prevention grants through SAMHSA. These grants have allowed us to fund community coalitions so they have the resources to implement local prevention programs. Rutland is one of our Partnership for Success communities. Through their grant, they are focused on underage drinking, binge drinking, and prescription drug misuse among youth. They work on underage drinking, partnering with local law enforcement. The grant also supports coalitions to promote information about proper storage and safe disposal of unused drugs, publicize safe drug drop-off locations and promote take-back events, encourage pharmacists to share specific cautions with patients when they pick up prescriptions for controlled substances, and encourage prescribers and dispensers to use the Vermont Prescription Monitoring System as part of their routine practice when they prescribe controlled substances.

Last year, the Health Department also received a grant from SAMHSA to expand early alcohol and drug abuse screening, brief intervention, referral and treatment services for adults over the next five years. The goal is to make this a part of the regular health care practice. In Rutland, the free clinic is one of those provider sites.

The Health Department administers both the SAMHSA block grant and Medicaid funds to support outpatient, intensive outpatient, residential, and medication-assisted treatment. We aim to ensure that everyone and anyone who needs treatment can access the right treatment as soon as possible.

With the opening of West Ridge in November and BAART Behavioral Health Services in the Northeast Kingdom in January, the State is implementing the Care Alliance for Opioid Addiction. The Care Alliance is a partnership of treatment centers and clinicians around the State using a hub-and-spoke model to offer medication-assisted therapy to Vermonters in need. The treatment centers, or the hubs, will serve patients with complex needs. Hubs offer comprehensive assessment and specialty treatment with methadone or buprenorphine, providing treatment much closer to home for many.

Connected with the hubs are the spokes—the Blueprint for Health practices and other primary care practices that treat patients using buprenorphine. Patient care at a hub or a spoke is supervised by a physician and supported by a network of community-based services aimed at our goal: enabling patients to be successful in life, work, and as family members. This system of care gives a health home for people addicted to opiates.

We also work closely with the criminal justice system to support both drug court programs and reentry services for people with addiction. To be effective, it is imperative that treatment services are tailored to people's specific needs. Clearly a person in the criminal justice system will need a different treatment regimen than a young mother who has just delivered a baby.

The Turning Point Recovery Centers are also supported with grants from the Health Department. We have 11 recovery centers around the State, including one in Rutland. The goal is to support all paths to recovery and to offer peer support to people who are trying to maintain recovery. The treatment centers work closely with the Turning Point Centers to ensure that clients make connections with peer support volunteers.

So there are a couple questions I wanted to specifically address that were posed to me. One, what do communities need to do to get ahead of the problem? In Vermont, we look to the evidence. Research has shown that a comprehensive approach using principles of effective prevention, intervention, treatment, recovery, and enforcement is most effective. Single-strategy approaches may solve one part of the problem or another, but will not hold up over the long term.

First, a community must make a comprehensive assessment to determine what their risk factors are. For example, before Rutland had acknowledged that they did not have an opioid treatment program, they had to acknowledge that and agree to create one. Getting to this point requires community education and discussion. Messages from key community leaders, like the mayor or the police chief, are key to raising community awareness.

Next, organize a group of community stakeholders to lead planning efforts. This group can establish goals and measures so that residents understand how the community is progressing in addressing this problem.

Finally, evaluate progress to ensure forward movement. As the saying goes, it truly does take a village of everyone working together to get ahead of the complex problem of opioid abuse.

What about preventing relapse and recidivism? Research shows that a person needs to be connected to treatment and recovery support for at least 90 days to get a firm foundation in recovery. It is important to have various levels of care available so that treatment can be tailored to individual needs. Some need intensive outpatient treatment, some need detox and residential care, stabilization and transition to outpatient care. Medication-assisted therapy, such as is provided through The Care Alliance for Opioid Addiction, is the evidence-based treatment indicated for opioid addiction.

Recovery services are essential for making new connections with people who do not use drugs. Changing one's environment is key to long-term recovery. This may mean getting sober housing, learning employment skills, whatever it takes to build a new life.

The Agency of Human Services works hard to ensure that comprehensive wraparound services are available to meet a client's needs. This is essential to preventing recidivism, and it is a priority of AHS.

Two recent national reports underscore that all three branches of State government are committed to finding solutions. A report from the Trust for America's Health commends Vermont's use of all 10 nationally recommended strategies to reduce prescription drug abuse and overdose. A National Safety Council report credits our State as one of only three to meet all of its standards on State leadership and action, prescription drug monitoring, responsible prescribing, and overdose education and prevention.

As we work to address the demand side of the equation, we cannot underestimate the power of prevention. We see hope and progress in the 2013 Vermont Youth Risk Behavior Survey results that shows use of tobacco, alcohol, and prescription drugs by Vermont youth declined since 2011—all priorities for our community-based prevention efforts. Investing early in the health of young people clearly yields the best return on investment.

Thank you, Senator Leahy and Representative Welch, for listening to this testimony on this important issue.

[The prepared statement of Dr. Chen appears as a submission for the record.]

Chairman LEAHY. Well, thank you. Thank you very much.

I should note, incidentally, that all of the statements of the witnesses will be in the record in full. And I should also point out that we have other statements—Joseph Kraus from Project VISION and from other law enforcement officers, EMTs, judges, education providers, and community members.

But I also want to note that we are doing this somewhat differently than we normally do. I find that sometimes the things that really get the most attention in the Senate are when somebody says, "Let me tell you a story," and I get specific stories. So I am inviting anyone listening to submit testimony to opioid ▮hearing@judiciary-dem.senate.gov. Or you can go on the Committee's Website, and up until this Friday we will take testimony or comments you might give. There are cards with that information in the back.

I have found that as technically adroit as I am with computers, I am usually brought up short, if not by my kids, by my grandkids. When a five-year-old asks to go on a particular Website, I say, "I will call it up for you"—you can hear me saying this, Chief, to get to the Website. My grandson takes the mouse out of my hand and says, "Let me take over because it gets very complicated."

[Laughter.]

Chairman LEAHY. So we have the information for submissions printed out on a card. I saw my staff going, "Don't try to explain it. Just give them the card" because the email address is complicated. But the point is that—and I will be sharing these with Congressman Welch—do send in your stories of things that worked, but also of things that did not work, because it is helpful.

Now, one thing that does work, I believe, is the Boys & Girls Clubs, and Mary Alice McKenzie is the executive director of the Boys & Girls Clubs of Greater Burlington. She has worked with a formal task force aimed at cutting off gang activity, working with members of law enforcement, and the child welfare community. Marcelle and I have gone by—I have lost count of the number of times we have gone by the Boys & Girls Clubs in Burlington. We have seen her take young people who many times because of where they live or who their families are could have been at great risk, and work with them to help them stay clear of drugs, to stay clear of addiction.

So, Mary Alice McKenzie, the floor is yours.

STATEMENT OF MARY ALICE MCKENZIE, EXECUTIVE DIRECTOR, BOYS & GIRLS CLUBS OF GREATER BURLINGTON, BURLINGTON, VERMONT

Ms. MCKENZIE. Thank you so much, Senator. I cannot tell you how grateful I am that you are holding the hearing today, grateful to Congressman Welch for being here to support this, and incredibly grateful that you asked me to testify to what I hope is to give voice to the interest of children. And I think in the discussion we are having in the State we love so much, the interest of children has not yet become the centerpiece of the discussion in the way the Boys & Girls Clubs around the State believe it should be. And so I want to thank you for allowing me to hopefully give voice to the interest of children, and in that regard, I also want to acknowledge that my colleagues from other clubs are here to give their support. Larry Bayle is here from the Rutland Club, Mike Reiderer is here from the Vergennes Club, and Beth Baldwin Page is here from the Brattleboro Club. And I want to thank them for taking the time——

Chairman LEAHY. Would the three of them please raise their hands so we can see where they are? Oh, great. Thank you very much.

Please go ahead.

Ms. MCKENZIE. Now, as you know, because you have been so good to all of us at the Boys & Girls Clubs around the State, we are all different. We are smaller than others. Some are bigger, some are smaller. We may serve slightly different age groups. But we have a common mission, and our mission is to "inspire and enable youth in our communities, especially those who need us most, to realize their full potential as productive, healthy, caring, and responsible citizens." And so although we may differ in our political views, the size of our communities, the way we deliver our services, we are in solidarity with each other on how to execute our mission, and we have all independently, quite frankly, concluded that because of what we are witnessing in our community around addiction, that we cannot not engage, because if we do not engage on pushing back on the trends that we see, we will violate our reason for being. So we have engaged in slightly different ways, but we have all engaged.

We agree with each other that the trends are really quite bad. The trends have gotten worse over the last decade. But we also believe that if we take coordinated and comprehensive community actions, we can make the difference.

And so we are doing different things based on what our community needs. In Burlington, we started getting very concerned about what we were witnessing in our neighborhoods about three years ago. We started seeing evidence of trafficking in a way that we had not seen in my lifetime. I am a native. I have lived in Burlington my entire life. I have never seen anything, never thought I was going to see what I have been seeing in the neighborhoods.

Most importantly, and of most concern, were the things that children were telling us. Now, at the Boys & Girls Club, we serve children from the ages of five through 19, so we truly are talking about children and youth. And we had children telling us that they were afraid to walk home at night, afraid to walk across the park, afraid to walk down North Street to their family apartment.

They told us being followed, harassed, and assaulted by those under the influence of drugs, 13- and 14-year-old children telling us that they had been approached by people who were living in their neighborhood to carry backpacks or to serve as lookouts; 15-, 16-year-old girls told us of being offered money for sex by the same people who were selling drugs in their neighborhoods.

We started having to make more and more reports to DCF about children who were being severely neglected because there was no food in the home, because there was no money left for food to feed these children.

We learned very disturbingly of access being made to middle-school-aged girls in exchange for drugs. We heard about guns, and we heard about gang affiliations.

Now, all of these things did not happen all at once. They were spread over a period of time, and we found ourselves making more and more reports. And then we looked around at ourselves, around the staff meeting table, and said, "We can make all the reports in the world, all of the mandated reports to the police, to DCF, to parents, and it is not enough." Simply making reports and expecting somebody else to fix the problem is not going to fix the problem. And so we started to dig in and trying to find out what could we do, what did we have control over, what actions could we take to make it better in our community. We reached out to a number of people in positions of authority and people who had access to edu- cational resources, because, after all, we are not the first commu- nity walking this path. Many communities have walked this path before.

We contacted Boys & Girls Club of America. They sent their director of delinquency and gang prevention to Burlington for three days to take a look at the situation, to do training, to leave us with educational materials and some tools that we could implement to try to get at how bad was the problem, because, quite frankly, we were not sure how bad the problem we were dealing with was. This was an invaluable source of help for us.

We were also made aware of a particular grant that could have helped us with some start-up funds. However, when we received the invitation to apply, we realized that we did not qualify because the grant was written for a much larger urban area. And so that was a disappointment, but rather than say, okay, well, we cannot do anything because we are underfunded, we reached back out to somebody more local. We reached out to the United Way and, in particular, Martha Maksym, who has been an absolutely incredible support for us. And together with the United Way, we decided we are doing two things: We partnered with Tris Coffin and his group around the opiate effect panels to educate our community about the problem, and we also started looking for flexible funding, which, thankfully, we were able to find, and so we used the money to contract and collaborate with Spectrum—again, a knowledgeable source, Spectrum Youth Services, in the business of treatment—to work with us to say what are the best practices. How do we create a culture of health as opposed to a culture of addiction? They are right in our backyard, and Spectrum and the Boys & Girls Club have said, you know, Boys & Girls Club, if you do not do your job well, addicted youth are going to end up with Spectrum, so let us come together and use what we both know to improve the chances for at-risk kids.

We also contacted the Burlington Police Department, and our incredible chief of police, Mike Schirling, was right there with training and educational services and resources for us.

Most important, we started listening to our kids in a very different way. We all have a tendency to lecture kids. We all have a tendency to tell them what they should do. I think often we do not just ask them, "What do you think? And what do you need?" We surveyed and we are still surveying our kids on a very methodical basis. We have held focus groups and panels, individual conversations. I myself have talked to hundreds and hundreds of kids, and they have told us a lot. They have told us, "If you talk to me in high school about drugs, it is way too late. I smoked or my friends smoked their first joint when they were eight or they were nine or they were 10"—pick a number. It is incredibly young. It is shockingly young.

"If you tell me, 'Just say no to drugs,' or if you tell me if I do drugs I am going to die, that is a joke to me, because I know people who bring drugs to school, they bring drugs to parties, they do drugs, and nobody I know has died yet. So do not just tell me if I do drugs I am going to die."

"If you only tell me about drugs when I am in health class in high school, that is also a joke to me, because it is a check-off-the-box exercise."

"If you think that I am serious, then treat me seriously," is what they are saying. They are saying, "Tell me the facts. Tell me what drugs do to my brain. What do drugs do to my looks? What do drugs do to my prospects? Give me the facts. Take me seriously."

These messages are coming from all different kinds of kids—rich, poor, middle class, natives of Vermont, from places far away—but they are common messages.

Now, there is a different set of messages and they are much more complex from the kids who are most at risk, who I believe and the rest of the clubs believe are in the minority. However, as we all know, the minority can affect the majority. These are children that we really do not talk much about because we do not know how to deal with them in Vermont. We all see the news when people are arrested here for trafficking drugs. They come here from the Bronx, Brooklyn, from Chicago, wherever. And we are mad, we are outraged that they bring these substances here and prey on the vulnerable. But what we do not talk about is that these people and people like them have been coming in and out of Vermont for a very long time, and they have extensive networks here, and they have relationships here, and they have borne children here, and their children and the children who are born into the households who are highly addicted are the most at-risk children in our community. And we do not have many tools in our toolbox for intervening early and effectively.

Unfortunately the only tool that we have had in our toolbox is to arrest and incarcerate when they reach a level of criminality that we can no longer ignore them. These are among the children who need us most, and we must confront this issue. And I do know that the issues are very complicated. They involve confidentiality rules and philosophies, prosecutorial, judicial, defense bar, legislative ideologies that are very uncomfortable to challenge. But we believe that we must address the needs of these children or they are going to be Vermont's next-gen inmates—something none of us want.

Thankfully the majority of our youth are not that complicated in figuring out how to help them. They have told us what they want. They want safe parks. They want safe streets. They want places to go on Saturday nights. They want more team sports. And they want clarity about the rules of health and safety.

At the Boys & Girls Clubs, we are listening. We have done soul searching. We have taken some actions. In Burlington, we have looked at our park across the street from our main site. There is a small, rundown storage building. We asked the mayor of our city if we could take it over. He said, "Absolutely. Bring it on." We found a private donor. We are taking the building over, renovating it, and turning it into an academic center. Not only will we be able to serve more kids more deeply, but we will improve the safety profile of the entire neighborhood.

We have adopted the United Way language around drug abuse and prevention, and we have adopted their goal, which is that all children and youth are free from addiction and its consequences, and we walk the talk, which is incredibly hard because walking the talk means that youth who you are trying desperately to save, if they continue to participate in illegal and destructive behaviors, then they have to be removed from the Boys & Girls Club. This is very hard to do. But we have done it. We have done it after a lot of soul searching. As a result, more youth are coming to us because they believe that we are going to provide safety for them.

We have increased our transportation capacity, so we are bringing kids home after dark if they need a ride. We have opened our club on Saturday nights. We have found more ways to get more kids in the club right after school, during the high-risk hours between three and six o'clock. We have increased all of our programming, including our academics and our team sports. We serve dinner six nights a week. It takes funding to be able to do this. We would not be able to do what we are doing without our board of directors, who also sees the challenges of addiction in the community and has said we must do what we must do. And so we will find the funding. We must find this funding to be sustainable, and we are not there yet on all the efforts, but we are resolved to getting there.

So some of these things are not rocket science. They are really boots-on-the-ground kind of actions. But we think that for our community, this is what is needed.

Now, every club is doing the same or similar things. In Rutland, Larry Bayle is actively participating with Project VISION.

Beth Baldwin Page is working with the local police in Brattleboro so that there is a coordinated response to any incident involving a child or youth.

In Vergennes, Mike Reiderer has long been known as a leader in delivering prevention programs.

There is also serious mentoring going on for other communities who want something like a club or a Boys & Girls Club. Larry Bayle is mentoring the communities of Randolph and Lyndonville right now because we all recognize that we individually and collectively have to do our part.

I think the good work that has been done so far is obviously early stage and, quite frankly, I think it is the easy work that has been done. The hard task is ahead of us, and that is creating a unified front on all fronts: prevention, intervention, including treatment, and suppression.

And I want to close by emphasizing one thing. I know that I have been talking about prevention measures and real boots-on-the-ground kind of strategies. But I have to say that coordinated and well-done law enforcement really, really matters. In Burlington, when the U.S. Attorney's Office, the federal agencies, Burlington Police under the leadership of Mike Schirling, all started working together, we noticed. Our neighborhoods did get more safe, and we have to remember that. It cannot all be on their shoulders. We all have to do our work. But we have to allow them to do their work, too, because without them, we do not have a chance.

So I want to thank you so very much for allowing me to testify.

[The prepared statement of Ms. McKenzie appears as a submission for the record.]

Chairman LEAHY. Well, thank you very much. You and I have had the privilege of being——

[Applause.]

Chairman LEAHY. You and I have had the privilege of going to some of the annual Boys & Girls Clubs breakfasts in Washington, DC, and I think, like me, you have been almost moved to tears, if not moved to tears, by some of the stories of young people who have turned their lives around with the help of the Boys & Girls Club and have now become such models in their community.

I have told this story many times, and I will tell it very briefly here. A number of years ago, we were trying to get some grants from the Department of Justice and back to Vermont, and I called a police chief of a small police department and said, "I think I can get you a grant for a couple more officers." He said, "Do you know what I would rather have?" And I said, "What?" And he said, "I would rather have a Boys & Girls Club." He said, "I do not need to arrest more kids. I need to have a place for more kids to go so they will not be arrested."

Really, that is what it is all about.

Colonel L'Esperance is a 27-year veteran of law enforcement in Vermont. In 2009, he was named director of the Vermont State Police. He has specialized in narcotics investigations, criminal highway interdictions, and worked extensively with the Vermont Drug Task Force, including as commander of the Criminal Division at State Police Headquarters. I can go through all the many accomplishments. He has a bachelor's degree in criminal justice from Champlain in Burlington.

Colonel, you are somebody I have called dozens of times when I have had questions on programs that might or might not work, so please, sir, it is all yours.

STATEMENT OF COLONEL THOMAS L'ESPERANCE, DIRECTOR, VERMONT STATE POLICE, WATERBURY, VERMONT

Colonel L'ESPERANCE. Thank you very much, Senator. If I could repeat verbatim what Mary said about prevention and treatment—excuse me, prevention and education, I would do that. I think that was the most compelling testimony I have heard about that, and I think that is the core of where we need to go.

Ms. McKENZIE. Thank you.

Colonel L'ESPERANCE. I would like to start by thanking Senator Leahy and Congressman Welch for the opportunity to appear before the Senate Judiciary Committee to address the many challenges that we are facing in Vermont related to heroin and opiate addiction. From a law enforcement perspective, the numbers are staggering. According to data provided by the Vermont Drug Task Force, in just the past two years alone, we have seen a 482-percent increase in the number of heroin investigations initiated by drug investigators and a 247-percent increase in the amount of heroin seized as a direct result of those investigations.

Instead of focusing on the numbers, however, I would like to use my time here to focus on the solutions. Heroin and opiate addiction is a very real and complex issue that requires a dynamic response from all the stakeholders involved. For every statistic cited about heroin there is someone behind it who struggles every day to either stay clean or seek out their next fix. There are no easy answers, but we can and we will make progress as long as we are united and determined. From a statewide perspective, we must combine all our efforts and resources to reduce those abusing opiates through treatment, stop the flow of heroin into the State with strong enforcement, and prevent another Vermonter from heading down the road of addiction through education.

I applaud Governor Shumlin for bringing this issue to the forefront in his recent State of the State address. As the director of the Vermont State Police, I will continue to strengthen our statewide enforcement efforts while building coalitions with our partners in treatment and prevention. Law enforcement must continue to disrupt supply lines that are responsible for bringing large quantities of heroin into Vermont and further work to prevent drug traffickers from getting a foothold in the State. I am pleased to say that I can report on a number of achievements we have made.

This past year the Vermont Drug Task Force conducted multiple high-level arrest sweeps across the State in Bennington, Springfield, and St. Albans. The primary goal of these operations was to dismantle heroin distribution rings operating within our communities and subsequently damaging our quality of life. I can say without hesitation that these operations were a success not only because we slowed the supply of heroin by arresting those responsible for distributing it, but because we were able to impact so many other lives in positive ways.

One such story came to me through the form of an email from a mother whose adult daughter had been struggling with her addiction. Her daughter was eventually arrested in the drug sweep in Springfield. It was clear from her email that she felt she had lost her daughter to heroin until the day she was arrested. She said unequivocally that her daughter's arrest ultimately saved her life. After the sweep, her daughter was able to break free from a bad relationship, get the necessary treatment she needed, and eventually reunite with her own young children. She expressed appreciation in her email to law enforcement for intervening at a time in her daughter's life when nothing else seemed to be working. There are many similar untold stories resulting from the work being done by the Drug Task Force. Each story has a positive message of appreciation, resolve and a commitment to taking the community back from drug dealers.

The Drug Task Force truly provides a specialized and valuable resource to State and local law enforcement agencies in our statewide efforts to reduce drug supply. Time and time again, the task force model proves to be one of the most successful management tools used by law enforcement today in Vermont and across the Nation.

In addition to the achievements of the Drug Task Force, I have been working with my command staff to implement a plan to issue naloxone to every trooper in the state. It is called Narcan as well. Having this drug in the hands of first responders will ensure that it is available, if necessary, to reverse the effect of a drug overdose that could potentially mean the difference between life and death. This is an important step to further our public safety mission and one that I am proud to support. We are working hand in hand with our Department of Health to ensure this process moves forward.

As a rural State, we face unique challenges in our efforts to curb drug abuse and the effects it has on our citizens. We do not have the luxury of the vast resources that exist in urban cities or suburban regions, so to be effective we must pool our resources and collaborate together in order to solve these problems. Although it can be more difficult to find solutions in a rural State such as Vermont, the fundamentals of illegal drug markets are the same everywhere. Where there is a demand, there will always be a supply. We cannot ignore this fact, and we must work to both disrupt drug trade and reduce demand. Commissioner Flynn is 100 percent focused on this issue.

This past January we invited Dr. William Roberts of the Northwestern Medical Center to speak to the entire command staff of the Vermont State Police about addiction. Dr. Roberts is a specialist in pain management and a leader in Vermont on addiction issues. I believe that forging these types of partnerships between law enforcement and the medical community is essential to breaking down barriers between the two groups and generating an intelligent and comprehensive approach to resolving this problem.

It is often said that law enforcement cannot solve this problem alone, but the truth is that no one can solve it alone. We must continue to build strong relationships like the one the Vermont State Police now has with Dr. Roberts at the Department of Health and Bob Bick of the Howard Center in our effort to drive down demand and ultimately reduce the influx of heroin into the State.

As we move forward, I will continue to rely on the tremendous support we have received and continue to receive from both the State and Federal Government. Without the funding secured by Senator Leahy over the years—and it does go back decades—our ability to operate the Drug Task Force at the level of success it enjoys today would not be possible. Subsequently our ability to positively impact local communities and rural sections of the State would be severely diminished.

With your help, we will continue to focus on our mission of preventing further abuse through education and outreach as well as reducing both the supply and demand of heroin through strong enforcement and an equally strong treatment response.

I would like to thank Senator Leahy, Congressman Welch, and the entire Committee for the opportunity to participate today. Thank you.

[The prepared statement of Colonel L'Esperance appears as a submission for the record.]

Chairman LEAHY. Well, thank you very much.

[Applause.]

Chairman LEAHY. I would also note that Jeff Unger of Senator Sanders' staff is here, too, and this is something that all three members of our delegation are trying to work very closely on, also with the Governor.

Let me ask the U.S. Attorney a question. You talked about—and it is a tragic case—going with the father of this young man who died to high schools and talking to students. And I think we all agree that the "Thou shalt not" kind of thing is not very effective. It has got to be a lot more than that.

What do you draw from those conversations? What do you feel gets across to the students?

Mr. COFFIN. I think it is really important for the students to have somebody that they can relate to, who they think is not trying to exaggerate or moralize to them. And one of the great things is Skip is just excellent at that. He was a math teacher for 30 years. He gets high school kids. He is very eloquent. And really I think the biggest message that people get is just the power of what he is saying. It is clear that this is something he carries with him every single day of his life. And for kids to see what that is like really opens their eyes. They see the film. The film has a lot of other people who—you know, Derek Hallquist did an amazing job capturing kind of this real straight, direct human stuff and this truth and honesty. And I think kids wake up to that and listen to that.

Chairman LEAHY. Well, do you get feedback on, "Well, that is somebody else. That does not affect me"? Or do they really ask questions?

Mr. COFFIN. Yes, a little bit. You get all kinds of response, and some of it is, "Oh, come on," a little roll of the eyes. But then when they think about it a little bit, you know, it is like a Russian roulette situation. It might not be you, but, you know, it was that guy. He is here to tell me about it, and it was him, and he started off taking a few pills and, you know, threw his whole life away. And there is this guy, he is doing a 16-year bit in federal prison. And it gets their attention.

Chairman LEAHY. I remember the pediatrician who spoke up in St. Albans at one of these hearings.

Mr. COFFIN. Dr. Holmes, yes.

Chairman LEAHY. Dr. Holmes, whom we all know well, and he explained to parents that opiate addiction was a real problem among people of the age of their daughter. And they said, "Well, we will certainly be watchful for this." He said, "You have not been watchful soon enough. I am talking about your daughter."

Mr. COFFIN. Right.

Chairman LEAHY. And I tell you, you could hear a pin drop in that room. That got everybody's attention.

There was a sentencing hearing, I am told, last week in federal court in Burlington, a young woman, conspiracy to distribute heroin and cocaine. She had been an addict for years. Can you tell me what was unique about that case?

Mr. COFFIN. Sure. You know, there are a lot of things unique it and a lot of things that were sort of an archetype. This was somebody who got wrapped up with a very violent and serious high-level drug trafficker, three prior drug convictions, selling a lot of heroin and crack, and she got herself involved where she was doing all those things for him to feed her addiction. You know, a victim of domestic violence and a lot of other really terrible exploitation by this person. But she got into federal court, and unfortunately a lot of terrible things have to go wrong for somebody to end up in our court. But when they get there, it is not always the end of the story. And we have got an amazing court and an amazing probation office, and when somebody goes through our court, they get assigned a case manager to follow them. They can get access to first-class drug treatment, supports, and other things they do to follow them through and get them on the right road.

And, you know, there is sometimes some tough love and there is sometimes some soft love, as the case goes on. And really what they do is they manage the case to make sure somebody does not fall off the path too far before they are pulled back onto it. And there are consequences for not complying, and there are rewards for complying. And this person was able, after some early slip-ups, to get into inpatient drug treatment, benefited greatly from that, maintained additional counseling throughout, urinalysis to make sure that she is really clean and not just hoping she is clean, and for eight months was able to remain clean and is on the right road. She is going to be under supervision by the same staff at the probation office for a period of time longer, but the sentencing judge was extremely pleased with that outcome.

And that is not a unique outcome. It is one that does not happen all the time, but it is far from unique, and I think it is important to recognize.

Chairman LEAHY. It is a lot better than warehousing in a prison.

Mr. COFFIN. Absolutely.

Chairman LEAHY. I am going to go back and forth on this. As I mentioned before, I was born in Montpelier, and that is a particular type of city. Then when I practiced law, I lived in Burlington, first in private practice, then as a prosecutor. I now live on a dirt road in the town of Middlesex, Vermont. I mention three really different communities.

So my question to Mary Alice McKenzie is: In Burlington, we have a Boys & Girls Club. What do you do in rural areas? My nearest neighbor is half a mile away. Now, the blessing of that is it is my son and daughter-in-law and an 11-year-old granddaughter. But what do you do in a rural area?

Ms. MCKENZIE. Well, we have talked a lot about this with the Boys & Girls Clubs, the group of us, and it is tough in a rural area. But I think you start with what you have got. You look at what are your assets in the community, what do you have for youth, and you build on what you have. Almost everybody has got a school. Almost everybody has got a school that has got a gym. Almost everybody has got caring adults, maybe college students. So you have got something to start with. And if the goal is find out what the youth lack and try to plug that gap, then you use what you have got.

Boys & Girls Clubs, however, do come in all shapes and sizes. There are some that are very tiny.

Chairman LEAHY. I know.

Ms. MCKENZIE. You know. And the key is to keep an effort sustainable, so be very realistic about what assets you have that you can use and what is the plan going forward so that you do not start something one year and then you are done the next year. That is doing a disservice with you.

As those of us who have mentored other communities say first and say very often, if you look to building a youth organization around public money, municipal budget money, you are going to fail. So the community has to support it, whether that is a $10,000-a-year support level or more than that.

So I think you start with what you have got and you build on that, and you make it sustainable. And I really think you can be a very small community and make that happen if you have the will to do it.

Chairman LEAHY. Speaking of communities coming together, I am going to ask Chief Baker this. I made a comment in the cloakroom off the Senate. Several Senators were talking, talking about what we are going to do during the recess, because the House and the Senate are out of session this week, and I said that Congressman Welch and I are going to be holding a hearing in Rutland, Vermont. They said, "Oh, the city that was on the front page of the *New York Times.*" I said, "The city is on the front page of the *New York Times* because they came together to address a problem. They came together because of a community response." And I said, "I guarantee you, every one of you has a Rutland in your State, but have they come together?"

So tell us a little bit about Project VISION. How has this helped in the turnaround?

Chief BAKER. Thank you for recognizing that, Senator. You know, we have had varying reaction to the media coverage we have here in the city over the last couple weeks, but many of us do take the same position you take, that we are there because we recognize we have this challenge. We recognize that the challenge is affecting the quality of life in our city. It plays out in family disturbances, neighborhood disturbances, acts of disorderly conduct, larcenies. And we recognize that the only way we are going to do this, as I said earlier, is all hands on deck.

I think one of the things when we started this conversation a couple years ago—and some of the testimony here today fits exactly what I am about ready to describe—many of us operated in our old silos. You know, we hear this all the time in law enforcement, that law enforcement has these turf battles, and we operate in silos, and we do not share information. You know, it is the same story that has been repeated over 20, 25, 30 years. What is real challenging— and I heard Mary Alice talk about this earlier—is when you start bringing in non-traditional partners and you want to share infor- mation and they play from a whole different set of rules than you do when it comes to sharing information, if I want to talk to an- other police officer about someone who may be dealing drugs, I meet him in a parking lot and grab a cup of coffee, and I say, "Hey, this is what I am hearing." Try to have that with someone who has a mental health crisis worker who has a patient on their caseload or a social worker or somebody in the medical field, because of reg- ulations around such things as HIPAA. It makes it very difficult to be able to have those conversations and break down those silos. The other thing that I think we found challenging is within those silos where there are only so many dollars on the table, and some- times the best intended people will fight over quarters that are lay- ing on the ground. And at the end of the day, I think what we have come to realize here in Rutland is fighting over those same dollars does not make sense.

So what we need to do is everyone can hold onto their own dol- lars, everyone can hold onto their own grants, but how are we going to collectively take that and set metrics and figure out how we are doing better, and how are we going to do that collectively. And I think that has been the most revealing, most challenging, but the most strength-building exercises we have done, are around those kinds of conversations we have had, where people have had to put aside what their traditional beliefs are about how to get to the bottom of this problem. And it has built unbelievable partner- ships, unbelievable relationships, and I will give you one example. Last Friday, the social workers that are housed inside our build- ing, dancing around the issues of confidentiality and making sure that, you know, we are not violating the privacy of other folks. A conversation broke out with one of the social workers that led us to realize that there were two registered sex offenders living inside a residence that we would not have known about if, in fact, we did not have those kind of conversations around the water cooler.

And I know when you came to visit us and we took you on the little tour upstairs, you know, I talked to you about the water cooler and the coffee pot. It is where it happens. It is where it happens. It is where we are finding out what is going on in our community that are putting members of our communities in harm's way, and the difference is because everyone is together, we are reacting to it collectively.

And I am happy to report—it is about 2:35 right now—that those two individuals were arraigned at one o'clock today on violations because of the sexual registry. And that would not have happened, Senator, if we did not have those kind of relationships.

Chairman LEAHY. And I agree, and they are important. And it is also important to not fight over the quarters but rather fight for a result. And I think when some of my colleagues hear what you had to say, you may get invites to come to other States and tell them how to do it.

Dr. Chen, I am not a medical person. I have heard that naloxone, which is used to counter the effects of an opioid overdose, and naltrexone, which blocks the high one might get and prevents relapses and can be administered every 30 days. Are these drugs good? Bad? Either? Both?

Dr. CHEN. Well, Senator, I think you have heard from Colonel L'Esperance about naloxone and it——

Chairman LEAHY. And he came in and briefed me in my office about that.

Dr. CHEN. It is a potentially life-saving drug and has a very— has a strong place in terms of harm reduction. So this past year, the legislature actually passed a bill in Vermont to both allow for naloxone to be administered, allowed immunity for people calling 911. So if you are using with somebody and they go down, you are able to call 911 without being afraid of being prosecuted. So it really has a place. It has a place in public safety vehicles. We have actually revised rules now in Vermont so it virtually can be carried in every ambulance that has an EMT on it. So those are all available.

Chairman LEAHY. So your department supports naloxone?

Dr. CHEN. Absolutely. But it is not a magic bullet. I think it needs to be part of a comprehensive approach, both in terms of prevention, intervention, and treatment.

In terms of naltrexone, that is a drug where we are investigating how we might use it. We all thought perhaps in the past that Antabuse might be a wonderful drug for alcohol abuse, we do not use it much, if at all right now. And I think that we need to find the appropriate place for this naltrexone. One place that it seems like it might make some sense is to interface and link with the correctional system. So you have an inmate who is coming out of the correctional system who may be at particular risk for using again, and providing them this drug with a strong commitment to enter into treatment and to enter into community supports, this might be a reasonable strategy for them. So we are actually—in a few weeks, I am going to meet with the manufacturer of the drug.

Chairman LEAHY. As you do, to the extent you can, can you keep me and my office and Congressman Welch and Senator Sanders posted on that, what you are finding?

Dr. CHEN. Absolutely.

Chairman LEAHY. And, last, Colonel L'Esperance, one of the things I found probably the most difficult choice when I was a prosecutor is when to withhold prosecution. It is always easy to say, okay, technically this is a violation, I will prosecute. But then there are times you ask youself, does somebody deserve a second chance or not?

You mentioned in your testimony, after one of the sweeps—let me make sure I have got this right. You were contacted by a mother who told the story of how her daughter's arrest ultimately saved her life. How do we make a determination when it is time to try an opportunity or a program that might give someone a second chance? Is there some automatic formula? Or does this really require a judgment call, one at a time?

Colonel L'ESPERANCE. I think, Senator, that working hand in hand with the prosecutor to understand the background of the individual that we are talking about. I think in the world of heroin, there are only two people that do not benefit from it: the poppy farmer himself and the addict. Everybody in between, there is a profit there. So we——

Chairman LEAHY. That is an interesting point.

Colonel L'ESPERANCE. We need to focus on those individuals. Jail is a place for someone that profits from heroin distribution. There is no two ways about it. Those individuals that are addicted that need treatment need to be recognized early on in the process, and I think there are a number of programs now that are there that do this. But to give someone a second chance is what we are here for, whether it is Narcan—I never thought I would need immunity to save someone's life, I will be honest with you. It was the easiest decision I have ever made as colonel. And the positive response from law enforcement across the State, and I hope that every squad room and every crew in the State eventually has that, because that individual that has overdosed, it takes them from the jaws of death and they have a mother, a brother, or father, an uncle that would love nothing more for a second chance.

Chairman LEAHY. You know, we have a man who is now chief of emergency services in a major metropolitan hospital who tells the story about being a young resident at the University of Vermont, and there was a place called "The Place" in Burlington, where people could come with an overdose. And these young residents and interns were volunteering their time. There was no law that said they could do it. I just said there would be no prosecution, and the police said they would not surveil it. The one thing is they had to empty their pockets, give any drugs they had, partly because we wanted to test the drugs and see if strychnine and other things were going in it. This doctor tells me he was a week away from graduation. He goes out to the State Police barracks out on 40th at the time with a big bag of drugs. He had a ponytail and a Fu Manchu moustache. He comes walking in with this bag saying, "Either this immunity"—which is not written down anywhere—"is actually going to work, or there goes how many years of medical training down the drain."

[Laughter.]

Chairman LEAHY. He hands it to the sergeant, and he said, "This was at The Place." He says, "Okay." Leaves it there. He said, "Do you want my name?" He said, "I do not want it. Leahy does not want it. Good-bye."

[Laughter.]

Chairman LEAHY. So talk about your immunity triggered that memory.

Peter.

Representative WELCH. Well, you know, that story that you just said reminded me of the great Gillie Godnick. We were in Rutland, and he said, "You know, Peter"—he educated me my first term in the Senate. He said, "Sometimes you got to forget about principle and just do the right thing."

[Laughter.]

Chairman LEAHY. That sounds like Gillie, rest his soul.

Representative WELCH. Dr. Chen, a couple weeks ago I was up at the Howard Center, the treatment program, with the drug czar and the Governor, and there are a lot of adults coming in there and getting the treatment on the way to work. And this problem that we are facing is affecting all ages, the kids, but a lot of adults. And one of the causes that a lot of us, I think, are hearing about is the prescription, some would say overprescription, of pain medication that people get for very legitimate reasons, but then find that the powerful effects of that are tougher than to stop taking it or looking for some alternative when the reason for the prescription has long since passed.

So the question I have is: What role is the medical community in the prescription of these powerful drugs playing in, adding to the burden? And what is it that we can do about that?

Dr. CHEN. So, Congressman Welch, your point is absolutely well taken. I think that the medical community does share responsibility in why we are all sitting here today. I think that if nothing else, the Governor's State of the State would certainly highlight for each and every physician who is practicing and prescribing in Vermont.

I think that we have strategies in place that can improve that, whether it be educating physicians about appropriate prescribing, educating prescribers to use the drug data base, the Prescription Monitoring System, to ensure that people are not doctor shopping and diverting drugs to creating a set of kind of guidelines and rules that would really be universal precautions so that when you do prescribe opiates for a person on a long-term basis, you want to ensure that you get informed consent so people know what they are really getting into and what the risks are. You want to make sure that they are being screened for potential substance abuse. And you want to make sure that they are agreeing to work with you, as a partner with a physician, whether it be urine tests to make sure they are taking the drugs or not taking other drugs, whether it be pill counts. All of those things, I think, are important strategies that medical providers could use.

And so right now we are working on some of those rules. I know in the workers' compensation bill are another set of rules that Vermont wants to use, even more stringent, as the "insurer" to ensure that both people get adequate treatment for their pain but they can get back to work sooner, because it is clearly shown that the more opioids they get, the longer it takes for people to get back to work.

Representative WELCH. Thank you, Dr. Chen.

Chief Baker, one of the challenges is how do you provide support to the person that is making the decision that they want to get off, and it has got to be tough for some parents whose kids have made the wrong choices here.

What are your dealings with parents? And is that something where there are ways with this broad-based approach that can help parents help their kids?

Chief BAKER. My experience personally here as the chief, as I talk about often between my career in the State Police and being here as chief, I am very close to the citizens in Rutland just by the nature of what my position is. Ironically, just today I got an email from a woman who I spoke to about 10 months ago who had a son who was addicted, and she emailed me today to tell me that her son was clean for about six months, and she was celebrating, as she said in her email, getting her son back.

Representative WELCH. But they need some support, too, right?

Chief BAKER. Absolutely. When you hear some of these stories from the parents who—you know, I do not know what this defini-tion is—did everything right, for all of us in this room that are par-ents, and you listen to these stories, it is heart-wrenching. And they just turn to anywhere they can to find help. And I do think that we are lucky we have some support groups in this community, but I think there has to be a way to support these folks that are fighting this with their kids. And, you know, they go to bed every night. You hear these conversations with these parents. They do not know where their kids are. They know they are abusing. They are going to bed. They are just waiting for that knock to come on the door. And to hear those stories over and over is heart-wrench-ing.

And I think much of this, we do not sometimes measure the re-sidual fallout from that for these parents, and I think it is abso-lutely crucial that communities create some space and be sup-portive of those folk that are going through it, because, you know, as the saying is, by the grace of God there go I. And, you know, it is heart-wrenching to hear these stories, and there is not a week that goes by—I have a woman who is waiting to hear from me now that wants to talk to me about her daughter who has been fighting addiction for over five years.

Representative WELCH. Thank you.

Mr. Coffin, I know that sentencing issues are really important federally, and I know quite a while ago Senator Leahy had Judge Sessions appointed to the Sentencing Commission with a lot of de-bate about whether the old-style sentences that are still current law are a hindrance or a help. And, obviously, you are on the front line in your current job as the U.S. Attorney here in Vermont. Do you have any thoughts about whether there is room for sentencing reform that would be useful?

Mr. COFFIN. Yes, definitely. I think a lot of the academic re-search shows that a shorter period of time that is certain to be im-posed is a greater deterrent than a longer period of time that is more of an uncertain consequence. And following up on that, Attorney General Holder has really charged us in a series of changes to how we charge our cases to look at more individualized assessments of each defender and their particular circumstances and their particular offense in determining what type of offense to charge, because in the federal system, and in other systems, too, the nature of the charges that the prosecutor brings can drive to a significant extent what the sentencing outcome is.

Also, Attorney General Holder has more recently, in some memos last August, directed us to limit our charging of mandatory minimums in cases where people are low-level, non-violent, and do not have serious criminal offenses. And I think those are really good changes, and, you know, one of the things I was lucky to be able to do. And our U.S. Attorney community nationally had some hand in crafting some of those changes.

Representative WELCH. Thank you.

And, Mary Alice, I just want to ask you, I have not been to the Boys & Girls Club as often as Senator Leahy, but I have been there, and it is an incredible place with lots going on—chaos in one area, people playing games, and then quiet in others where people are studying. It is really quite remarkable.

But with those kids who are there versus you see kids who come in from all kinds of different families, some intact, others not, what are the things that the community can do that give the kids and the parents of those kids the best shot of having those children make better choices?

Ms. McKENZIE. Well, I think adults can start acting like adults, take responsibility for their kids. It does not matter what kind of background. Kids are like sponges, and they pick up the messages. And if you tell them on the one hand do not do drugs, but they see you on the other hand drinking a lot, using a lot of marijuana, they are not going to believe you. And it does not matter whether they are the most at-risk kid or a secure kid, because the path—kids that get into trouble, it is a really pretty similar path. They early are exposed to some addictive substance, seeing it in action. They try it. They go to a home where there is no adult in attendance, and they try it. Some are going to be okay. Others are not going to be okay. And those that are not going to be okay go up the chain of addiction. And you see it over and over and over.

And so I think that as adults, if we accept our responsibility for the health, safety, and well-being of our children, then we all need to walk the walk.

Representative WELCH. Okay. Thank you.

Colonel L'Esperance, I was with Senator Leahy this morning, and he reminded me, in response to a question, about our highway fund, that we spent 42 trillion in Iraq, and he was wondering, you know, that money might have been spent in other places.

Chairman LEAHY. Like the U.S.

Representative WELCH. Well, the point here is that it is a tough time in Congress right now on budget and fiscal issues. But, on the other hand, it is a tough time in communities facing real challenges that need a partnership, and the partner should be federal tax dollars, which are your tax dollars, being wisely used to help communities that are willing to help themselves. And you mentioned that the Drug Task Force approach, which you have a lot of experience with, in your view—and, of course, Chief Baker, you too—has really been effective. So, you know, this is the person both on Appropriations and Judiciary that probably has as much influence as anybody, short of the President. What is your message to us to bring back to our colleagues about the value of funding these drug task forces, the COPS grant, and the Byrne grants?

Colonel L'ESPERANCE. I think if you speak to the chiefs and sheriffs behind me, they could tell you themselves. The funding at the local level, State level, when that gets diminished, we depend so heavily on—on Senator Leahy in particular—federal funding. I was the envy of my colleagues across the country for a number of years when we had a way of getting money to Vermont, so we were very fortunate. The Drug Task Force was built, the foundation of the task force was built on federal funding. But it became a house of cards after a period of time. But there is State legislation that Senator Sears in particular has supported and directed to the task force, and the chiefs and sheriffs behind me that buy into this, they send officers into the task force now with no funding backup. They understand the significance. It goes beyond the boundaries of their community.

Representative WELCH. Okay. Thank you.

Colonel L'ESPERANCE. Thank you.

Representative WELCH. Thank you very much.

Chairman LEAHY. I want you to know that there is now an effort to go back to doing things in Appropriations where we actually care about some of the needs here in this country. I think you are going to be happy that is going to happen. I am also going to try to reauthorize very soon the Leahy bulletproof vests bill.

[Applause.]

Chairman LEAHY. As we close, one thing. The mayor has been here through the whole hearing—and, Mr. Mayor, thank you very much because you have been very, very good at working with us on this, and I thank you for that. We have here the Attorney General, our Attorney General, our U.S. Marshal, and so many others in law enforcement.

And, last, this is the card.

[Laughter.]

Chairman LEAHY. So that I do not have to have one of my grandkids tell you how to do it, take that card. If you have some testimony you want to give, please limit it to 10 pages and get it to us by March 21st.

And I mention this, think about it, if you have something you want to say, whether you agree or disagree—agree or disagree—feel free to do it. You know, we put testimony in the record, like Sheriff Marcoux's and others, but this is going to be a part of the permanent record in the U.S. Senate. Both Republicans and Democrats will be influenced on this, on the question. And I will make sure the Appropriations Committee will see it, too. We do go by seniority in both Committees, and as some have heard me say, as I said earlier this morning, when I came to the Senate I had no seniority, and I hated the system; but now that I understand it——

[Laughter.]

Chairman LEAHY [continuing]. Having studied it for a few decades, I love the system. And they will hear about it.

And I want to thank Peter Welch. He has got 40 different places he is supposed to be today, and he has been so concerned about this issue. He has been a great partner over in the House. The two of us have tried to approach this as a non-partisan issue. I have joined with some of the most conservative Republicans in the Senate as well as some of the most liberal Democrats, and we have been effectively able to get legislation through.

This is not a political issue. This is our children. These are our family members. These are our brothers and sisters. In some instances, this is our parents. Let us work together. I think you know that we will be there for you because you have always been there for us.

We stand in recess.

[Applause.]

[WHEREUPON, AT 2:58 P.M., THE COMMITTEE WAS ADJOURNED.]

APPENDIX

Witness List

Hearing before the
Senate Committee on the Judiciary

On

"Community Solutions to Breaking the Cycle of Heroin and Opioid Addiction"

Monday, March 17, 2014
Franklin Conference Center at the Howe Center
1 Scale Ave., Rutland, VT 05701
1:00 p.m.

The Honorable Tristram Coffin
U.S. Attorney, District of Vermont
Department of Justice
Burlington, Vermont

James Baker
Chief
Rutland City Police Department
Rutland, Vermont

Dr. Harry Chen
Commissioner
Vermont Department of Public Health
Burlington, Vermont

Mary Alice McKenzie
Executive Director
Boys & Girls Clubs of Greater Burlington
Burlington, Vermont

Colonel Tom L'Esperance
Director
Vermont State Police
Waterbury, Vermont

PREPARED STATEMENT OF CHAIRMAN PATRICK LEAHY

**STATEMENT OF SENATOR PATRICK LEAHY (D-VT.),
CHAIRMAN, SENATE JUDICIARY COMMITTEE
HEARING ON
"COMMUNITY SOLUTIONS TO BREAKING THE CYCLE OF HEROIN AND OPIOID ADDICTION"
RUTLAND, VERMONT
MARCH 17, 2014**

This hearing of the Senate Judiciary Committee will come to order. Today, we will examine the issue of heroin and opioid addiction, and how communities such as Rutland can successfully come together to solve this complex problem. This is a knotted complex of challenges that reaches into neighborhoods and communities of all kinds and sizes, in urban and rural areas alike.

Vermont has not been spared. Between 2000 and 2012, treatment for opioid addiction in Vermont rose by more than 770 percent. This is consistent with findings that the supply of opioids, including heroin, is expanding across the country. We have all heard the awful stories of young lives cut short by heroin overdoses. Vermont is ahead of most of the country in many ways: Our state has openly identified the problem, and we are all constructively seeking ways to not just help addicts get clean, but to stop this scourge in its tracks. We have heard it many times, but it bears repeating: We cannot arrest our way out of this problem. Prevention, education, and treatment must go hand-in-hand with the important efforts of law enforcement.

Many eyes are now on Vermont. Governor Shumlin has spoken forcefully about the heroin crisis. Its impact is so significant that he dedicated his State of the State message to the problem this year. The Chief Justice of Vermont, Paul Reiber [RYE-ber], has added his voice in the search for solutions, noting in a recent speech: "This challenge is complex and cannot only be met with the blunt tool of criminalization." Opioid addiction is an issue of great importance to me, not just as a Vermonter, but as someone who cares deeply about making sure we are developing real, lasting solutions. We need to get ahead of addiction and the corrosion that it brings into individual lives, families, and our communities.

As Chairman of the Senate Judiciary Committee, I work to solve problems in our criminal justice system at the federal level. What I have seen is that when we look for creative solutions, when we want to find ways to save money and make smart changes, we often look to the states for fresh ideas.

States are often the incubators of innovation. When we in Washington see what's working in the states, we can adopt that approach for the federal system. Vermonters do not shy away from a challenge. True to form, we have developed some innovative programs in our state by pooling community resources to most effectively help our citizens. Here in Rutland, Chief Baker is working collaboratively with Mayor Louras, residents, community developers, housing advocates and prevention specialists, and is making real progress in identifying ways to break the cycle. This community response, known as Project VISION, serves as a model for how neighbors can marshal forces to confront the drug and related crime problems that plague their neighborhoods. Project VISION's director, Joe Kraus, summed it up this way: "We have two choices here. We can curse the darkness, or we can light a candle, to quote an old saying."

We know Rutland is just one example of how communities around Vermont are working together to confront this crisis. And we know that this challenge is not unique to Vermont's largest communities. Lamoille County Sheriff Roger Marcoux, in his written testimony for today's hearing, noted that roughly half of Vermont's opioid-related overdoses since 2011 have occurred in rural settings. So let us focus our efforts on all Vermont communities, big and small.

This is the fourth time in the past six years that I have brought the Senate Judiciary Committee to Vermont to explore issues related to drug abuse and its impact on communities. And although there continue to be challenges, I am hopeful as I sit here today. We often talk about a three-tiered approach to addiction: prevention, treatment, and enforcement. This combination forms the foundation for sound solutions. But Vermont has shown that even more success is possible when these traditional roles are shared – when prevention, treatment, and law enforcement are not separate efforts at all.

I learned from my years as State's Attorney in Chittenden County how important these collaborative efforts are. And today I see a law enforcement community that, more than ever, is fully committed to prevention and treatment efforts. Law enforcement would rather not arrest and prosecute the same offenders over and over when the underlying issue is a treatable addiction. Treating the addiction can be the better and less costly approach. It has the added benefit of fewer cases landing on detectives' and prosecutors' desks.

One of the programs I am working on in Washington is the Second Chance Act, which I have introduced for reauthorization and hope to bring before the Senate Judiciary Committee soon. This program supports initiatives like the Vermont Court Diversion Program, which allows offenders charged with minor crimes to keep their record clean if they successfully complete a program designed for them by community review boards.

I applaud the innovative diversion models that have emerged in response to community needs, such as Windsor County's Sparrow Project and the rapid intervention efforts in Chittenden County. These programs effectively divert substance abusers from the courts to treatment providers. They have shown very promising results in easing court caseloads, reducing recidivism, and moving addicts towards recovery. These are just a few examples of how communities are working together to identify solutions.

Our witnesses today have devoted much time and energy to breaking the cycle of addiction in our communities. Vermont's U.S. Attorney, Tris Coffin, has taken his message of prevention into Vermont schools, along with the father of a University of Vermont student who died five years ago from a heroin overdose. They relate how addiction hurts not only addicts, but their families, friends and neighbors. Chief Baker is facilitating a community-based response, and his message is clear: Not on our streets; not in our town. Dr. Chen, with his years of experience as an emergency room physician, is working with Governor Shumlin to take the prevention message to our communities and to our schools. Mary Alice McKenzie is working through the Boys & Girls Clubs to respond to the needs of our kids, who want to have positive, healthy, and supportive alternatives to addiction. And the Vermont State Police, under the direction of Col. L'Esperance, and in partnership with the Vermont Department of Health, are using a promising drug, naloxone [nah-LOX-own], which can immediately reverse the effects of a heroin overdose. This initiative has the potential to not just change the dynamic between law enforcement and the communities they serve, but to save lives.

Vermont has recognized that heroin and opioid addiction is not a problem our small state can ignore. The lessons we have learned here in Vermont are important for the whole nation. I look forward to hearing from all of you working to improve your communities and end the cycle of addiction.

I want to thank Congressman Welch for being here today, for the day an honorary member of this panel. I know he, too, is concerned about this cycle of addiction. I want to also thank the many people here in the audience today. You represent law enforcement and our judicial officers; you are our health professionals and our recovery experts. Here today are education providers and students, civic leaders, veterans and representatives from youth organizations. Government, from the federal, state and local levels is represented here. Everyone here today is the embodiment of this community-minded approach to breaking the cycle.

As a Vermonter, I thank everyone gathered here today for your commitment and dedication to addressing this thorny and complex problem. And as a Vermonter, I'm proud of the ways that we come together to do what needs to be done.

#####

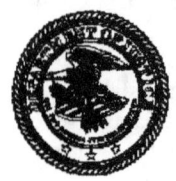

Department of Justice

STATEMENT OF

TRISTRAM J. COFFIN
UNITED STATES ATTORNEY
DISTRICT OF VERMONT

BEFORE THE

COMMITTEE ON THE JUDICIARY
UNITED STATES SENATE

AT A FIELD HEARING IN RUTLAND, VT

ENTITLED

"COMMUNITY SOLUTIONS TO BREAKING THE CYCLE OF HEROIN
AND OPIOID ADDICTION"

PRESENTED MARCH 17, 2014

TESTIMONY OF TRISTRAM J. COFFIN

BEFORE THE UNITED STATES SENATE

COMMITTEE ON THE JUDICIARY

March 17, 2014

Thank you for bringing the Senate Judiciary Committee to Vermont and for inviting me to share with you my views about the need for a broader community reaction to heroin and other opioids trafficking, use and addiction. I, and the Department of Justice, appreciate your leadership on these issues for so many years, and your dedication to improving the lives of Vermonters.

First let me say that Rutland is a terrific small city. It has a strong and proud community and a great tradition. But it is a community, like many others throughout New England and the United States, that is going through a difficult time right now. Many communities are having to face up to the many significant challenges that are presented by opioid trafficking and addiction. Rutland is addressing these problems in a forthright, aggressive and creative fashion. I commend Chief Baker and the rest of the Rutland community for doing that.

The heroin and opioid problem in Vermont is not new. It has been building for some time. Under your leadership, this Judiciary Committee has held three field hearings in Vermont on the issue of drugs including opiates in prior years. As the problem of opioid addiction began to emerge, you invited Attorney General Holder here for the Opiate Prescription Medication and Heroin Summit we held in September 2010. As was stated in that hearing, the problem existing then of rampant addiction to opioid prescription medications would soon lead to rampant heroin trafficking and addiction in Vermont. And indeed that has happened.

On March 10, 2014, Attorney General Holder, in a public video message, called the rise in overdose deaths from heroin and other prescription pain-killers an "urgent public health crisis." I couldn't agree more. The numbers and statistics are stark. Between 2006 and 2010, heroin overdose deaths increased nationally by 45 percent. Heroin treatment numbers are up over 250% since 2000 and over 40% in the past year. Our office's prosecution of heroin traffickers is up, with indictments more than doubling last year and totaling more than four times what they were just a few years ago. To me, one of the starkest statistics is the increase in fatal heroin overdoses here in Vermont. Last year's total, twenty one, was more than twice as many as the year before, and five times the number of just five years ago. These are extremely concerning numbers. I want to echo the Attorney General and urge first responders to carry the drug known as naloxone. When administered quickly and effectively, naloxone immediately restores breathing to a victim in the throes of a heroin or opioid overdose. I applaud the Vermont State Police and the Vermont Health Department for moving forward on this issue. When you deal with the families of overdose victims who are left behind, I can tell you that every one of these numbers has a face and a name, and loved ones left behind in pain that does not go away.

The Justice Department, along with our partners in the Vermont State Police and the Rutland Police Department, have been aggressive about prosecuting traffickers who seek to profit out of selling this misery. And we will continue to do so. But what this hearing is about is how important it is for the community to respond as a whole to this problem. We will remain active and vigilant on the law enforcement side, but it is not enough. This problem requires a broad community response, and I am thrilled that under the leadership of Chief Baker and others, Rutland is engaged in making this response. And similar, other broad community responses to this problem are happening throughout other parts of Vermont as well.

Attorney General Holder has been very clear with me and my fellow U.S. Attorneys that we need to be smarter on crime, not just tougher. We are not giving the community what it deserves if we offer up only an expensive solution – unlimited incarceration – that does not address the root causes of the problem. When we look at the problem of heroin and opioid use, law enforcement alone is not sufficient to address the problem. Community responses emphasizing prevention and treatment are essential complements to work in conjunction with law enforcement to make the community safer and more drug free.

Over the last three years, I have been fortunate to be involved in one such prevention program. On March 23, 2009, Skip Gates lost his treasured son Will to a heroin overdose. Will was an outstanding young man. He was in his third year at the University of Vermont, studying molecular genetics, a standout alpine ski racer, an incredible young man. We met Skip through the investigation of the heroin trafficker who sold Will the heroin that led to his death. Skip was searching for some way to turn this tragedy into something positive. Working with our office's outstanding crime victim advocate and a great young filmmaker named Derek Halquist, Skip had the courage to share his personal experience of this tragedy in a short film, the Opiate Effect.

We sent the film to all the high schools in Vermont, for free, two years running. For the last three years, Skip and I have traveled throughout Vermont, playing the movie and speaking to young people and parents about the dangers of opioid use. Skip is an eloquent speaker, and the film is powerful. I think a lot of the power of the movie comes from its informational approach. Young people see firsthand the impact heroin has had on Skip, and on his family. They hear from recovering addicts straight talk about what life as a heroin addict is like. The film doesn't moralize. Rather, it lays out the real facts on what life as an opioid addict is all about so young people can make clear choices. In this way the film moves the conversation beyond "just say no."

The film has been well-received throughout Vermont and has won several awards. We've also set Skip up with the U.S. Attorney's Office in Maine where he has done similar work in his home state. We've tried to push the film out nationally and it is available for a free download.

The importance of this, of course, is to try to stop people from entering the opioid addiction and criminal justice pipeline. Because once that happens, there are no good outcomes. Only varying degrees of bad ones.

That is why the prospect of effective drug prevention is so important. We do a lot of work to reduce the supply of drugs coming into this State. But if we are not equally as aggressive on reducing the demand side, our efforts will be of little avail. We need better and more drug treatment to get people who are addicted to these substances off of them. And we need better and more comprehensive prevention approaches to reduce the number of people who fall into this trap. Law enforcement is not the only answer. We need these other efforts as well.

To be successful, these prevention and treatment efforts must come from broad segments of the community. Like those occurring in Rutland and Burlington and many other communities in Vermont, we need to have realistic discussions of the issues communities face from opiate and other substance abuse, and look to the ingenuity and creativity in these communities for newer, broader solutions. We need to ask ourselves what we can do to better educate kids and parents so we reduce drug use at an early age. What can we do to give kids better things to do than to be exposed to drugs? What can we do to divert people from entering the criminal justice system? What can we do better to treat those addicted and get them on the right road? What can we do to help neighborhoods not be comfortable places for drug traffickers?

And when we have these discussions, we need to understand that comprehensive approaches, rather than piecemeal or solely law-enforcement oriented measures, are necessary to solve the problem. Comprehensive solutions rooted in the community, and tailored to each community's unique situation and characteristics, solutions that draw upon the perspectives, skills and insights of a variety of stakeholders – not just the police.

The other witnesses today I know have much to add on this score, so I will close my remarks. But let me do so by thanking the Chairman for permitting me to speak today on behalf of the Department of Justice, and for his substantial, dedicated and caring leadership on this issue over many years.

TESTIMONY OF CHIEF JAMES W. BAKER

BEFORE THE UNITED STATES SENATE

COMMITTEE ON THE JUDICIARY

RUTLAND, VT

17 MARCH 2014

Senator Leahy and members of the Senate Judiciary Committee, on behalf of Mayor Chris Louras, Mr. David Allaire the President of Board of Alderman, elected officials of Rutland City government, members of the Police Commission, the citizens of Rutland, and the men and women of the Rutland City Police Department, welcome to the City of Rutland, Vt. We are proud of this great City and we are honored you have taken the time to bring a field hearing to us to learn of the good work being done here to address the challenges of substance abuse and in particular opiate abuse.

I want to echo the comments of U.S. Attorney Tris Coffin that the City of Rutland is a terrific community with a strong and proud history. This hearing is being held in a building that is representative of Rutland's proud history. This building dates back to the 1800s when the Howe Scale Company, was based here. After years of productive output, Howe Scale fell on hard times and the company closed in the early 1980s leaving this expansive manufacturing complex, with more than 330,000 square feet, vacant. What to do with this vast structure soon became the source of intense public debate and disagreement.

The debate about the future of the Howe Center has been captured and memorialized. It serves as a reminder of the challenges Rutland has faced. It serves as a reminder of the grit of this great city. Just as Rutland created a new vision for the Howe Center, we are committed to remaking Rutland into one of the healthiest and safest cities in the United States. In fact, the Vision Statement of Project VISION is:

Reclaiming Rutland: Healthiest, safest and happiest community in America!

We have the people, the infrastructure and the will to get it done.

Not unlike other communities, the city of Rutland has faced the challenges of illegal drug activity before. In the early 1990s, as a young supervisor of a multi-agency drug task force, I worked out of Rutland and was involved in countless undercover drug operations that resulted in arrests, prosecutions and convictions for drug distribution. The drugs of choice were cocaine and marijuana. At that time, I was convinced that the resources and efforts we applied had solved the drug problem in Rutland. Fourteen years later, I became the Director of the Vermont State Police and Rutland City Police Chief, Tony Bossi, sought help from the State Police with a new and emerging drug problem. The call for help was based on the fatal shooting on Grove Street during a drug deal and reports of violence involving firearms. The city had reached the tipping point on drug activity and violence. After a significant commitment of resources, a drug sweep rounded up more than 40 defendants in an operation known as *Operation Marble Valley*. The cases had strong out-of-state influences marked with a serious presence of gun culture and the drugs involved were cocaine, crack cocaine and heroin. At the press conference announcing the arrests, officials made the point that these arrests were meant to change the direction of the drug culture in Rutland.

Around the same time under Senator Leahy's leadership, a U.S. Senate Judiciary Committee field hearing was held in this very room. There was testimony about the need for prevention, treatment and enforcement. The community rallied for a period of time.

In January 2012, I arrived in Rutland as the Interim Chief of Police to find there was yet another emerging drug challenge. This time the drug was heroin. I found a police department that was demoralized and a community who had no trust in the police department. The dispirited atmosphere stemmed from the fact that there was an unrealistic expectation that the police department could and should single handedly resolve the issues of illegal drug trafficking. As more pressure was applied to the police department to act, the more aggressive the law enforcement actions became. The measure of success was the number of arrests made and the amount of drugs seized. The trouble with those success measures was that history clearly showed that arrests alone were not going to change the environment because it does not take into account the underlying social issues relating to drugs. Not one of the underlying issues that lead to addiction is under the control of the police, yet the solutions to the issue were laid at the door step of the police department. It became apparent that in order to affect change in our escalating drug crisis; a crisis from our experience that originates at its base from initial addiction to prescribed medications, the situation was going to require all hands on deck.

As we began the conversation with our non-law enforcement partners, we worked to gather a coalition of local, state, county and federal enforcement partners to change the culture and environment on the street by employing laser-focused enforcement operations. That effort resulted in *Operation Fedup* and was coordinated by ATF and our others partners. The first operations seized nearly 8,000 bags of heroin and approximately $90,000 in cash. That investigation led to the connection of a drug distribution network in New York City. The furtherance of the investigation under the guidance of U.S. Attorney Coffin, the DEA and FBI, revealed an organization that was responsible for up to 10,000 bags of heroin coming into the Rutland area on a continual 10-14 day basis. It was hard to fathom the depth of the addiction in this area that would require that amount of heroin. It was a shock to all. This was the first epiphany. We could no longer follow the methods deployed in the past if we were to move the ball down the field. The demand for opiates was outstripping our ability to be effective.

The second epiphany came tragically on September 26, 2012 at about 6 PM on Cleveland Ave in the City of Rutland. It was on that day that we lost one of our bright and upcoming stars. Carly Ferro, age 17, was leaving her place of work and entering into her father's car to ride home when she was killed. Carly was killed when a car operated by an individual, who is alleged in court papers to have been huffing aerosols, lost control of the car and struck her. The incident represented yet another critical point in Rutland's history where the grit and determination of her people was defined. This tragedy became a rallying point – a painful realization that what was happening in our city had to stop. The human costs were too high.

The non-traditional partners we had assembled became focused on creating metrics to measure where we were, and where we needed to go. We began meeting on a regular basis and followed a path modeled and championed by Chief Mike Schirling in Burlington known as Community Intervention Team (CIT). The vision was to join together all the resources available and create a multiplier force to affect the quality of life in Rutland. We brought to the table social service agencies, elected officials, police resources, the domestic violence advocacy community, drug court, corrections, prosecutors at the federal, state and local level, economic development officials, housing coalition officials, the faith community, mediation services, neighborhood citizens and many others.

In the early stages, the group talked and worked on strategies to create metrics using data to measure what success looked like. We worked on supporting and advocating for a methadone clinic. We worked on systems to better communicate across traditional and nontraditional partners. The energy was amazing.

The final epiphany came when Senator Leahy's staff located a grant opportunity from the U.S. Department of Justice Bureau of Justice Assistance. Our coalition refocused and developed a grant application that created the name Project VISION (Viable Initiatives & Solutions through Involvement of Neighborhoods). The grant created a blue print using outcome based modeling that we are following to execute our strategy.

We did not receive the grant. We think our good friends at BJA may have gotten this one wrong! However, we did not give up. The grit and determination of Rutland shined once again and we moved forward. We continued to execute our strategy and we now have an operating structure in place. We have stayed faithful to the concept of utilizing research to validate our processes.

Project VISION serves as an umbrella group that coordinates the functions of three committees. Those committees are Crime and Safety, Substance Abuse, Prevention and Treatment and Neighborhoods and Housing. Each committee is working on unique goals to their individual committee with the understanding that they stay faithful to Project VISION's key values of collaboration for the greater good and renewed focus on the positive.

As result of the collaboration of resources the Rutland City Police Department is now host to a variety of nontraditional partners who operate on the guiding principle that the issues we face associated with substance abuse, mental health issues and quality of life in our neighborhoods are interconnected. That interconnection requires an integrated response.

Today, housed in the Rutland City Police Department building, we have two social workers from the Rutland County Family and Children Center, a domestic violence advocate from the Rutland County Women's Network and Shelter, an Assistant Attorney General, an emergency crisis intervention specialist from Rutland County Mental Health, the Rutland County Early Intervention Coordinator, a School Resource Officer, Animal Control Officer, a Crime Analyst and a City of Rutland Building Inspector. These resources are coordinated by Captain Scott Tucker, the newly named Executive Director of Project Vision and the Commander of the newly formed Community Outreach Division.

In the police department we are embracing data and technology to identify where we apply these coordinated resources; never missing an opportunity to do case review, create systems of better communication and providing focused prosecution for those causing the most harm to our community. This effort coordinated daily, is brought together on a bi-weekly basis when all committee members attend mapping meetings. In the mapping meetings we look at the locations and the individuals that are causing the most harm. Based on that data, we develop integrated solutions to address each of those individual situations. As an example, in many of these cases the underlying issue of substance abuse and or mental health issues have led to family violence or neighborhood unrest. By having all the resources at the table, we can develop a response that includes more than the police response. This methodology influences better prosecution for proven offenders. Unlike in the past, police suppression is not our first or only choice. We are working at root cause issues.

It is important to note that we do still support and apply aggressive law enforcement to deal with those who choose not to meet our community norms and do serious harm. As an example, the sources of heroin that make a conscious decision to come to Rutland to deal need to understand that their behavior is not going to be accepted or tolerated. That is why we work closely with the Vermont Drug Task Force and our federal partners to apply enforcement resources. We pay close attention to those who choose to do harm in the form of violence against women and children, not accepting that addiction is the cause.

To demonstrate the determination of this great city I would ask anyone in the room who is associated in any way with Project Vision to please raise your hands. These are the faces of determination.

As I close, I want to thank all those partners who have worked to make our story worthy of telling in front of this committee. There are too many to mention, but you know who you are.

Honorable members of the Senate Judiciary Committee, thank you for being here today to take testimony. Senator Leahy, I thank you for your unwavering support for the City of Rutland. It is appreciated by all of us who are working tirelessly to get this right.

Thank you.

PREPARED STATEMENT OF HARRY CHEN, MD

Community Solutions to Breaking the Cycle of Heroin & Opioid Addiction

TESTIMONY

Harry Chen, MD, Commissioner of Health

March 17, 2014

Senate Committee on the Judiciary

Franklin Conference Center at the Howe Center

Rutland, VT

Vermont brought the problem of addiction to heroin and other opioid drugs to national attention this year. The numbers that quantify addiction as a public health crisis are startling for our small state: More than 50 Vermonters die from opioid drug poisoning every year. Deaths from heroin doubled from 2012 to 2013. Nearly 4,000 are in treatment for opioid addiction, and over half are young adults. More are waiting for treatment.

Vermont's experience has become the talk of the nation, for good reason. If it can happen here, in a mostly rural state made up of close-knit communities, blessed with natural beauty, where health care is nearly universal, with residents recognized as being among the healthiest of Americans – it can happen anywhere.

From my viewpoint, addiction must be recognized as a public health problem, and treated as a chronic illness. Addiction results from bad decisions, just like any of us might make to overeat or not exercise. But it quickly moves from a bad decision to disease. The end result is a chronic medical condition with profound implications for the individual and society.

That's why Vermont is taking a comprehensive public health approach to the problem of substance abuse and addiction – that involves prevention, early identification and intervention, an array of treatment services, and recovery supports.

It is now well accepted by that we can't simply arrest our way out of the problem. A bill passed last week by the Vermont Senate would divert non-violent drug offenders from being locked up in the criminal justice system, and instead get them into treatment as soon as possible.

And addiction is not someone else's problem – it's our problem. As a longtime former resident and doctor in the Rutland area, I, along with just about every other parent of young adults, know several of their classmates who were well-adjusted kids with caring parents whose lives were taken over by the horrors of opiate addiction. Thankfully, nearly all are now in recovery and doing well.

With the opening of West Ridge Addiction Treatment & Recovery Center in November 2013, we marked a milestone in Rutland County and for our state. We now recognize addiction as a chronic illness, like diabetes and heart disease, requiring a similar approach to prevention and treatment. We believe we are on the right path.

Let me describe our path in a little more detail.

The Vermont Department of Health has prevention consultants in each of our 12 district offices, including Rutland. Their role, as local experts, is to educate community members, help organize prevention efforts, and support coalitions with technical assistance to help implement proven prevention strategies.

We are fortunate to have a series of prevention grants through the Substance Abuse and Mental Health Services Administration (SAMHSA). These grants have allowed us to fund community coalitions so they have the resources to implement local prevention programs.

Rutland is one of our *Partnership for Success* communities. Through their Health Department/SAMHSA grant, they are focused on underage drinking, binge drinking and prescription drug misuse among youth – behaviors most linked to the greatest risks for youth. Their work on underage drinking involves partnering with local law enforcement.

Using guidelines provided by the Health Department, the grant also supports coalitions to promote information about proper storage and safe disposal of unused drugs, publicize safe drug drop-off locations and promote take-back events, encourage pharmacists to share specific cautions with patients when they pick up prescriptions for controlled substances, and encourage prescribers and dispensers to use the Vermont Prescription Monitoring System as part of their routine practice when prescribing controlled substances.

Last year, the Health Department also received a grant from SAMHSA to expand early alcohol and drug abuse screening, brief intervention, referral and treatment services for adults over the next five years. The goal is to make this a part of regular health care practice. Rutland Free Clinic is one of the provider sites that will become part of this pilot project.

The Health Department administers both federal Substance Abuse Prevention and Treatment Block Grant funds from SAMHSA and the state Medicaid funds, along with other funds that support outpatient, intensive outpatient, residential and medication-assisted treatment. We aim to ensure that anyone who needs treatment can access the right treatment as soon as possible.

With the opening of West Ridge in November, and BAART Behavioral Health Services in the Northeast Kingdom in January, the State is implementing the Care Alliance for Opioid Addiction. The Care Alliance is a partnership of treatment centers and clinicians around the state using a Hub & Spoke model to offer medication-assisted therapy to Vermonters in need.

Simply put, the treatment centers, or Hubs, will serve patients with complex needs. Hubs offer comprehensive assessment and specialty treatment with methadone or buprenorphine, providing treatment much closer to home for many. Connected with the Hubs are the Spokes – Blueprint for Health and primary care practices that treat patients using buprenorphine.

Patient care, at a Hub or a Spoke, is supervised by a physician and supported by a network of community-based services aimed at our goal: enabling patients to be successful in life, work and as family members. This system of care gives a health home for people addicted to opiates.

We also work closely with the criminal justice system and support both drug court programs and reentry services for people with addiction. We do this in partnership with the Court Administrator's Office and the Department of Corrections. To be effective, it is imperative that treatment services are tailored for people's specific needs. Clearly a person in the criminal justice system will need a different treatment regime than a young mother who has just delivered a baby.

The Turning Point Recovery Centers are also supported with grants from the Health Department. We have 11 recovery centers around the state, including one in Rutland. Their goal is to support all paths to recovery and to offer peer support to people who are trying to maintain recovery. The treatment centers work closely with the Turning Point Centers to ensure that clients make connections with peer support volunteers.

Another SAMHSA grant that was recently awarded to the Turning Point Centers' Recovery Network will allow them to place part-time staff with each Care Alliance Hub (in Rutland, that's the West Ridge Center) to focus on peer recovery and support.

What do communities need to do to get ahead of the problem? In Vermont, we look to the evidence. Research has shown that a comprehensive approach, using principles of effective prevention, intervention, treatment, recovery and enforcement, is most effective. Single strategy approaches may solve one part of the problem, but won't hold up for the long term.

First, a community must make a comprehensive assessment to determine what their risk factors are. For example, before Rutland had effective treatments in place for opioid addiction, they had to acknowledge that this was part of the problem and agree to bring evidence-based treatment to the community. Getting to this point requires community education and discussion. Messages from key community leaders, such as the Mayor and Police Chief, are key to raising community awareness and garnering support.

Next, organize a group of community stakeholders to lead planning efforts. This group can establish goals and measures so that residents understand how the community is progressing in addressing the problem.

Finally, evaluate progress, update goals and strategies, and report out to ensure forward movement. This also allows the community to see what progress is being made. As the saying goes, it truly does take a village of everyone working together to get ahead of the complex problem of opioid abuse.

What does it take to prevent relapse/reduce recidivism? Research shows that a person needs to be connected to treatment and recovery support for at least 90 days to get a firm foundation in recovery. It is important to have various levels of care available so that treatment can be tailored to individual needs. Intensive treatment is usually needed in the early stages so that a client can be stabilized first. That means detox if necessary, a short stay in residential care if they need stabilization, and then transition to outpatient care either with or without medication, depending on the substances they are abusing. Medication-assisted therapy, such as is provided through The Care Alliance for Opioid Addiction, is the evidence-based treatment indicated for opioid addiction.

Recovery support services are essential for making new connections with people who do not use drugs. Changing one's environment is key to long-term recovery. This may mean getting sober housing, learning employment skills, whatever it takes to build a new life. The Agency of Human Services works to ensure that comprehensive wraparound services are available to meet a client's needs. This is essential to prevent recidivism – and it's a priority of the Agency of Human Services.

* * *

Two recent national reports underscore that all three branches of state government are committed to finding solutions.

A report from the Trust for America's Health commends Vermont's use of all 10 nationally recommended strategies to reduce prescription drug abuse and overdose.

A National Safety Council report credits our state as one of only three to meet all of its standards on state leadership and action, prescription drug monitoring, responsible prescribing, and overdose education and prevention.

As we work to address the demand side of the equation, we can't underestimate the power of prevention. We see hope and progress in the 2013 Vermont Youth Risk Behavior Survey results that shows use of tobacco, alcohol and prescription drugs by Vermont youth declined significantly from 2011 – all priorities for our community-based prevention efforts. Investing early in the health of young people clearly yields the best return on investment.

PREPARED STATEMENT OF MARY ALICE McKENZIE

Testimony of Mary Alice McKenzie
Before the United States Senate Committee of the Judiciary
Rutland, Vermont
March 17, 2014

Thank you very much, Senator Leahy, for holding this very important Vermont field hearing of the Senate Committee of the Judiciary. This is indeed a critical time in Vermont because, as Governor Shumlin has bravely and publicly declared, we are facing serious challenges related to addiction and its consequences.

I am Mary Alice McKenzie the Executive Director of the Boys & Girls Club of Burlington. I am very grateful for this opportunity to testify about community actions we are taking in response to our challenges. I am most grateful for be given the chance to address the work being done in the interests of our most precious Vermont resource: children. The interests of children have not received enough attention in the Vermont discussion. And yet, it is a sad truth that children are often the first, and certainly are the most innocent, victims of addiction.

I and my colleagues, the Executive Directors of the other five Boys & Girls Clubs in Vermont, in Rutland, Brattleboro, Washington County, Vergennes and Randolph firmly believe that while addiction trends are bad, we CAN reverse them through comprehensive and coordinated actions. We believe that if Vermonters individually and collectively commit to actions that are unequivocally anti-addiction as well as anti-crime we can reduce the number of children who suffer the consequences of adult bad acts and poor choices.

The Boys & Girls Clubs in Vermont together serve thousands of Vermont children and youth from ages 5 to 18 every year. And although we differ from each other in certain ways, we share an identical mission to "inspire and enable youth in our communities, **especially those who need us most**, to realize their full potential as productive, healthy, caring and responsible citizens". We share the view that we violate our mission if we do not actively engage in pushing back against addiction lures and against those who make money exploiting the vulnerable and causing harm to children. We are remarkably uniform in our responses to Vermont's addiction problem not because we are similar in our political views or ideology. Rather, it is because we are all witnessing the abuse, the neglect, the damaged prospects of children that come as a consequence of addiction and drug related crime. The commonality of experience has caused us to acknowledge our role and responsibility in the fight for the well-being of the children who need us most.

In Burlington we sounded the alarm after seeing tangible evidence of increased drug trafficking impacting children in elementary, middle and high school grades. Kids began telling us that they were afraid to walk home after dark. Kids were followed, harassed and in a few cases assaulted by people under the influence drugs. Thirteen and fourteen year old kids confided that they or their friends had been offered money to sell drugs. Some fifteen year old girls told us that they had been offered money for sex by people who were also selling drugs. We were told about guns being carried by people dealing drugs. We became aware of situations where children were neglected because there was no money left for food. We learned that access to middle school aged girls had been given in exchange for drugs. We started seeing and hearing about gang affiliations. We, of course, made all the required reports to parents, police and DCF. But we also quickly realized that what we were experiencing was unlike anything we had seen before and that simply making required reports and expecting others to fix the problem was futile.

However, let me be very clear that good, coordinated law enforcement really matters. Without the coordinated, consistent work of the US Attorney's office combined with the resources of the Federal Agencies and the Burlington Police Department, the situation in our community would be far worse. And when those organizations started working very visibly together the community became visibly more safe. In addition, because of the leadership of Chief Michael Schirling, we often now get notice when arrests have been made in households where there are children. Sometimes, police officers will bring children directly to us so that the children are surrounded by support. Law Enforcement matters and while we must accept our own responsibility for action, we know that we will fail if law enforcement does not receive the support and the resources to do its' job.

In order to find out what we should do, we reached out to a wide range of people in Burlington. We invited schools, other youth serving organizations, DCF case workers, law enforcement officials, parents, landlords and others to a series of meetings. We learned that what we were seeing in our neighborhoods and what kids were telling us was being seen by many others. We also learned that many feared giving voice to the problem of drug addiction and drug related crimes. Some worried that going public would tarnish Burlington's reputation. Some feared that talking openly would set off a chain reaction of prejudice, discrimination and profiling. Others feared being discounted as just one more social do-gooder looking for a handout of public money. We were afraid too but took action anyway.

Some actions we have taken show success and some have failed. I would be happy to answer questions about failed actions. But for purposes of this testimony, I am going to focus on what has shown positive signs. Please understand that we are still finding our way through this and we certainly do not have all the answers, we are learning.

We reached out to and received help from Boys & Girls Club of America, specifically from Joe Mollner, the Director of Delinquency and Gang prevention programs at BGCA. A former Commander in the St. Paul Minnesota Gang Prevention Unit, Joe has a wealth of experience and a personal philosophy that we should never give up on any child. Joe came to Vermont for a three day review and assessment of our situation involving drugs, gangs and youth. He taught us how to survey our youth effectively. He also trained us in the methodology being used around the country to better serve and protect youth from the consequences of addiction and crime. The methodology involves a three pronged approach of prevention, intervention and suppression. Joe also gave us an invitation to apply for a specific grant that would have provided some funds to create a case management intervention program specifically designed for the most at risk youth. Unfortunately we had to decline that opportunity because the grant parameters, while appropriate for larger urban areas facing these same issues, were inflexible and unresponsive to our problems in Burlington, Vermont.

After the BGCA training help, we started to create forums for letting the kids tell us about what they were experiencing and about what they think they need from us. We have now surveyed and had group and individual conversations with many youth. And while there are some differences in what kids have told us, there are some very important consistent messages that are guiding us in the development of our actions. The consistent messages include:

"If you first start talking to me about drugs in high school, you are way too late. I smoked my first joint at (pick a number) from 8 to 12 years old."

"If you tell me in high school to "just say no to drugs" or that if I do drugs I will die, I won't listen to you. I know kids who bring weed or pills to school and/or to parties and no one I know has died yet."

"If you only lecture me about drugs in health class in high school, that is a joke to me because it's like just checking off the boxes of "healthy habits" so one day it's don't do drugs, the next day it's how to cook a healthy meal."

"If you are serious about me, treat me seriously, give me the facts, tell me what drugs do to my brain, tell me how to stay safe when I go to the party, because I will be at the party."

These are some common messages from kids who are rich, poor and middleclass. They are of different races, religions and from different places. There are, of course, different messages from the minority of kids who are already involved in heavy using. They are the smaller number of kids who are already into making money by stealing and dealing. They are the minority but unfortunately they influence the majority.

I must speak for a moment about the complexity of some of those youth, those who are at high risk of becoming Vermont's future inmates. We see and read about people from Brooklyn, the Bronx, Detroit, Chicago when they are arrested here for trafficking. We are outraged, and rightly so, that these people come here to sell products that cause such harm. What we do not discuss is that some of these same people have been coming here for a long time. They have extensive local networks and relationships here. They have born children here, children who are at very high risk. Like other communities, we must develop strategies to identify and intervene earlier and more effectively in the lives of these children. Very complicated issues exist here. Issues of confidentiality and of legislative, prosecutorial, judicial and defense bar philosophies. However, if we do not address this uncomfortable reality, our only recourse will remain arrest and incarceration when these youth reach a level of criminality that can no longer be ignored.

Thankfully, helping the majority is not quite as complicated. The majority want us to do more to keep them safe. They want to come to our sites more at night but they want to make sure they do not have to walk home after dark. They want the parks to be safe. They want to go to safe spaces on Saturday nights because the alternative is the streets, the parks or at homes where no adults are present. They want more team sport opportunities of all kinds. Often kids don't get to play on school teams and so their options are limited. They want us to be clear about the rules of safety, drugs and alcohol.

We have listened, done a lot of soul searching and taken the following specific actions:

We reached out to the City and requested approval to take over a storage building in the center of the park so that we can create a new teen and academic center. This enables us to deliver more focused academic support and will create a safer park. This relationship with the City is just pure positive, we have a donor who believes in this project and has agreed to do the renovations, we have our amazing Chief of Police Mike Schirling actively supporting our plan, and we have a Mayor who really understands the power of community partnerships.

We are working very closely with The United Way of Chittenden County to find resources and relationships to create more effective prevention strategies and to educate our community about the realities of drugs, addiction and crime. One of the goals of the United Way is that "all people are free from substance abuse and its consequences". The United Way is making connections all over Chittenden County to educate people who may think that addiction is someone else's problem. Because of the United Way's outreach efforts many now realize that addiction has an economic impact, a health care impact, an education impact, as well as a human impact that harms all of us.

Also, with the support of the United Way, we were able to find some flexible funding that is allowing us to create prevention strategies directly responsive to the needs of the kids we serve.

We have contracted with Spectrum Youth Services to develop the best policies, practices and culture for promoting health for a full range of children and youth of all ages.

We have adopted the language of the United Way and confirmed to kids that our goal is that "all youth are free from substance abuse and its related consequences". We have explained to the kids that the Club is a health and safety zone. And we walk the talk. This has meant some emotional tough times for us because we have had to take action to remove the few who engaged in illegal or destructive behaviors. We offer help many times and in many ways. But if the behaviors continue, the youth cannot be with us. Hard as suspending a youth from coming to the Club is, as a result, the total number of youth coming to us has increased because more feel comfortable coming through our doors.

We have expanded our transportation capacity and our hours of operation. We now are open on Saturday nights for teens. We have also started our own basketball teams with a goal of being able to participate in the Burlington league next year. We have expanded our music programing for teens. We have expanded our academic programs for teens such that they can come to the Club right after school instead of waiting until the evening hours. We serve dinner now six nights a week. All these things were things we could do in direct response to what kids told us.

Obviously, these efforts must be funded. Our board is a tremendous strength for us and when they saw our growing challenges, they agreed that we had to take whatever action we could to keep more kids more safe. Together, we re-prioritized where we could and increased our fund raising goals when we had to. We are pushing forward with resolve to make our efforts sustainable. It will take time but we all know that failure is not an option.

Every Boys & Girls Club in Vermont is working hard to help in their communities. Larry Bayle at the Rutland Club is actively partnering with Rutland's very impressive Project Vision, helping in many ways to support youth living in hard hit areas of the City. Beth Baldwin Page at the Brattleboro Club is working with law enforcement to create coordinated responses to incidents involving youth. The Vergennes Club, specifically Mike Reiderer, has long been a recognized leader in the delivery of effective prevention programs both in the Club and in schools. Kreig Pinkham at the Washington County Youth Services Bureau Boys & Girls Club manages many direct service programs to help youth in need. In addition, there are serious efforts to mentor communities who have expressed interest in forming a Boys & Girls Club. For example, currently Larry Bayle is mentoring the communities of Randolph and Lyndonville as they form Boys & Girls Clubs.

And while much is being done, we know that we are only at the beginning. The actions we have taken are good but much better work must be done. The hard task now is to create a united front, on all fronts, if we are serious about sustaining an environment of health and safety for our children. As adults, we must accept our responsibility for reversing our trends. We must work together to find the financial, political and human capital needed for prevention, intervention (including treatment) and suppression of addiction and related consequences. All Vermont's children, especially those who need us most, depend on us to get this right.

PREPARED STATEMENT OF COL. THOMAS L'ESPERANCE

U.S. Senate Judiciary Committee Field Hearing
Chairman, Senator Patrick Leahy
Vermont's Battle Against Heroin And Opioid Addiction
Monday, March 17, 2014
Rutland City, Vermont

Prepared Testimony – Colonel Thomas L'Esperance

I would like to start by thanking Senator Leahy for the opportunity to appear before the Senate

Judiciary Committee to address the many challenges we are currently facing in Vermont related

to heroin and opiate addiction. From a law enforcement perspective the numbers are

staggering. According to data provided by the Vermont Drug Task Force, in just the past two

years alone we have seen a 482% increase in the number of heroin investigations initiated by

drug investigators and a 247% increase in the amount heroin seized as a direct result of those

investigations.

Instead of focusing on the numbers however, I would like to use my time here to focus

on the solutions. Heroin and opiate addiction is a very real and complex issue that requires a

dynamic response from all the stakeholders involved. For every statistic cited about heroin

there is someone behind it who struggles every day to either stay clean or seek out their next

fix. There are no easy answers but we can, and we will make progress as long as we are united

and determined. From a statewide perspective we must combine all our efforts and resources

to reduce those abusing opiates through treatment; stop the flow of heroin into the state with

strong enforcement; and prevent another Vermonter from heading down the road of addiction

through education.

I applaud Governor Shumlin for bringing this issue to the forefront in his recent State of the State address. As the director of the Vermont State Police I will continue to strengthen our statewide enforcement efforts while building coalitions with our partners in treatment and prevention. Law enforcement must continue to disrupt supply lines that are responsible for bringing large quantities of heroin into Vermont and further work to prevent drug traffickers from getting a foot hold in the state. I am pleased to say that I can report on a number of achievements we have made.

This past year the Vermont Drug Task Force conducted multiple high level arrest sweeps across the state in Bennington, Springfield and St. Albans. The primary goal of these operations was to dismantle multiple heroin distribution rings operating within our communities and subsequently damaging our quality of life. I can say without hesitation that these operations were a success not only because we slowed the supply of heroin by arresting those responsible for distributing it, but because we were able to impact so many other lives in positive ways.

One such story came to me through an e-mail from a mother whose adult daughter had been struggling with addiction. Her daughter was eventually arrested in the drug sweep in Springfield. It was clear from her e-mail that she felt she had lost her daughter to heroin until the day she was arrested. She said unequivocally that her daughter's arrest ultimately saved her life. After the sweep, her daughter was able to break free from a bad relationship, get the necessary treatment she needed and eventually reunite with her own young children. She expressed appreciation in her e-mail to law enforcement for intervening at a time in her daughter's life when nothing else seemed to be working. There are many similar untold stories resulting from the work being done by the Drug Task Force. Each story has a positive message of appreciation, resolve and a commitment to taking the community back from drug dealers. The Drug Task Force truly provides a specialized and valuable resource to state and local law enforcement agencies in our statewide efforts to reduce drug supply. Time and time again the task force model proves to be one of the most successful management tools used by law enforcement today in Vermont and across the nation.

In addition to the achievements of the Drug Task Force, I have been working with my command staff to implement a plan to issue Naloxone to every trooper in the state. Having this drug in the hands of first responders will ensure that it is available, if necessary, to reverse the effect of a drug overdose that could potentially mean the difference between life and death. This is an important step to further our public safety mission and one that I am proud to support.

As a rural state, we face unique challenges in our efforts to curb drug abuse and the effects it has on our citizens. We do not have the luxury of the vast resources that exist in urban cities or suburban regions, so to be effective we must pool our resources and collaborate together in order solve these problems. Although it can be more difficult to find solutions in a rural state such as Vermont, the fundamentals of illegal drug markets are the same everywhere. Where there is a demand, there will always be a supply. We cannot ignore this fact and we must work to both disrupt drug trade and reduce demand.

This past January I invited Dr. William Roberts of the Northwestern Medical Center to speak to the entire command staff of the Vermont State Police about addiction. Dr. Roberts is a specialist in pain management and a leader in Vermont on addiction issues. I believe that forging these types of partnerships between law enforcement and the medical community is essential to breaking down barriers between the two groups and generating an intelligent and comprehensive approach to resolving this problem.

It is often said that law enforcement cannot solve this problem alone, but the truth is that no one can solve it alone. We must continue to build strong relationships like the one the Vermont State Police now has with Dr. Roberts in our effort to drive down demand and ultimately reduce the influx of heroin into the state.

As we move forward I will continue to rely on the tremendous support we have received, and continue to receive from both the state and federal government. Without the funding secured by Senator Leahy over the years our ability to operate the Drug Task Force at the level of success it enjoys today would not be possible. Subsequently, our ability to positively impact local communities and rural sections of the state would be severely diminished.

With your help, we will continue to focus on our mission of preventing further abuse through education and outreach as well as reducing both the supply and demand of heroin through strong enforcement and an equally strong treatment response.

I would again like to thank Senator Leahy and the entire committee for the opportunity to participate in today's hearing.

QUESTIONS SUBMITTED BY SENATOR GRASSLEY FOR JAMES W. BAKER

Senate Judiciary Committee

"Community Solutions to Breaking the Cycle of Heroin and Opioid Addiction"

March 17, 2014

Questions for the Record from Ranking Member Charles E. Grassley

James W. Baker, Chief of Police, Rutland , VT

1. In your testimony, you describe a joint law enforcement effort called *Operation Fedup*, which resulted in the seizure of over 8,000 bags of heroin. Were any other drug types seized in this operation? If so, please provide the other drugs and quantities seized.

2. In addition to heroin, what other illegal drugs are being distributed in the Rutland community? What do you estimate are the quantities of those other drugs being distributed and how do those quantities compare to heroin?

3. Do you believe that fully legalizing recreational marijuana, as Colorado and Washington states have done, would have a positive effect on Vermont's efforts to combat the crisis in opioid abuse?

Senate Judiciary Committee

"Community Solutions to Breaking the Cycle of Heroin and Opioid Addiction"

March 17, 2014

Questions for the Record from Ranking Member Charles E. Grassley

Dr. Harry Chen, Commissioner of Health, Vermont Department of Health

1. How many people are currently being treated for heroin or other opioid abuse in Vermont? How does that number compare to other illegal drugs? Is it accurate that in Vermont, more teens enter treatment with a primary diagnosis for marijuana dependence than all other illicit drugs combined?

2. Is there a relationship between the increased abuse of prescription opioids and the increased use of illegal opioids, such as heroin? If so, please describe that relationship.

3. What percentage of Vermont residents who end up addicted to opioids or heroin, or who seek treatment for such an addiction, begin their illegal drug use with, or also abuse, marijuana?

4. You mentioned in your written testimony that you "see hope and progress in the 2013 Vermont Youth Risk Behavior Survey results that shows use of tobacco, alcohol, and prescription drugs by Vermont youth declined significantly from 2011 – all priorities for our community-based prevention efforts." Is reducing marijuana use among youth also part of your community-based prevention efforts to battle opioid abuse? If not, should it be? What are the trends in the use of marijuana among Vermont youth from 2011 reflected in this survey?

Senate Judiciary Committee

"Community Solutions to Breaking the Cycle of Heroin and Opioid Addiction"

March 17, 2014

Questions for the Record from Ranking Member Charles E. Grassley

Mary Alice McKenzie, Executive Director, Boys and Girls Club, Burlington, VT

1. You mentioned that you have learned from youth in Burlington that there needs to be a consistent message provided to them about the dangers associated with drug use, even from an early age. As you wrote in your prepared testimony, kids have told you and your organization: "If you first start talking to me about drugs in high school, you are way too late. I smoked my first joint at (pick a number) from 8 to 12 years old."

   Do you believe that an important part of the community's prevention efforts to battle opioid abuse should include discouraging youth from using all kinds of illegal drugs, including marijuana? How has the recent debate over legalizing marijuana affected the ability of groups like yours to transmit a consistent message along these lines?

Senate Judiciary Committee

"Community Solutions to Breaking the Cycle of Heroin and Opioid Addiction"

March 17, 2014

Questions for the Record from Ranking Member Charles E. Grassley

Colonel Thomas L'Esperance, Director, Vermont State Police

1. In addition to heroin, what other illegal drugs are being distributed in Vermont? What do you estimate are the quantities of those other drugs being distributed and how do those quantities compare to heroin?

2. Do you believe that fully legalizing recreational marijuana, as Colorado and Washington states have done, would have a positive effect on Vermont's efforts to combat the crisis in opioid abuse?

Senate Judiciary Committee

"Community Solutions to Breaking the Cycle of Heroin and Opioid Addiction"

March 17, 2014

Questions for the Record from Ranking Member Charles E. Grassley

James W. Baker, Chief of Police, Rutland , VT

1. In your testimony, you describe a joint law enforcement effort called *Operation Fedup*, which resulted in the seizure of over 8,000 bags of heroin. Were any other drug types seized in this operation? If so, please provide the other drugs and quantities seized.

    There were no other drugs seized in that particular operation.

2. In addition to heroin, what other illegal drugs are being distributed in the Rutland community? What do you estimate are the quantities of those other drugs being distributed and how do those quantities compare to heroin?

    In Rutland we see crack cocaine as the second most distributed drug followed closely by the theft and diversion of prescription drugs. Those prescription medications are often redistributed on the black market.

3. Do you believe that fully legalizing recreational marijuana, as Colorado and Washington states have done, would have a positive effect on Vermont's efforts to combat the crisis in opioid abuse?

    I do not support the legalization of marijuana. I see clear defining lines between decriminalization, legalization and the retail sale of marijuana. It is one matter to have civil violations for possession of marijuana and another to legalize and sell marijuana on the retail market. The challenges as a police chief in the area of diversion of pharmaceutical drugs leaves me concerned that we cannot in fact regulate and control the distribution of marijuana.

    As to the impact of legalization of marijuana on opioid abuse, it is our experience that within the culture of the heroin distribution networks, the use marijuana is common. So common in fact that the probable cause developed for a good majority of traffic stops that result in the seizure of heroin, is often the presence of burnt and/or marijuana in the vehicle. As an example, our agency just seized approximately 400 bags of heroin and $8,000

in cash after responding to an active domestic violence call in the City of Rutland. Upon being greeted at the door of the residence the responding officers could smell a strong odor of burnt marijuana. This odor was the basis for further investigation that resulted in the arrest of New York City based individuals (who have extensive records) for trafficking heroin in Rutland, Vt.

To summarize, I do not see a positive impact if marijuana is legalized as it is in Washington and Colorado.

RESPONSES OF DR. HARRY CHEN TO QUESTIONS SUBMITTED BY SENATOR GRASSLEY

Senate Judiciary Committee
"Community Solutions to Breaking the Cycle of Heroin and Opioid Addiction"
March 17, 2014
Questions for the Record from Ranking Member Charles E. Grassley
Dr. Harry Chen, Commissioner of Health, Vermont Department of Health

1. How many people are currently being treated for heroin or other opioid abuse in Vermont? How does that number compare to other illegal drugs? Is it accurate that in Vermont, more teens enter treatment with a primary diagnosis for marijuana dependence than all other illicit drugs combined?

   In fiscal year 2012, nearly 3,500 individuals were served by state-funded providers for opioid abuse or dependence in Vermont. More youth under the age of 18 are treated for marijuana than for all other substances combined. Please see the below tables for details.

Number of people treated in the Alcohol and Drug Abuse Programs Treatment System by substance of abuse and year, Vermont

Substance	2000	2001	2002	2003	2004	2005	2006	2007	2008	2009	2010	2011	2012
Alcohol	4715	4997	5063	4997	4987	4743	4866	4696	4510	4358	4112	4176	4061
Marijuana/Hashish	1066	1286	1377	1596	1466	1567	1623	1571	1388	1563	1432	1430	1365
Heroin/Other Opiates	399	599	767	1041	1199	1455	1897	2113	2272	2630	2622	2944	3479
All Others	351	353	402	482	495	624	699	835	713	567	522	549	517
Total	6531	7235	7609	8116	8147	8389	9085	9215	8883	9118	8688	9099	9422

Data Source: Vermont Substance Abuse Treatment Information System (SATIS)
This reflects only people receiving treatment at state-funded treatment facilities.

Number of people under 18 years of age treated in the Alcohol and Drug Abuse Programs Treatment System by substance of abuse and year, Vermont

Substance	2000	2001	2002	2003	2004	2005	2006	2007	2008	2009	2010	2011	2012
Alcohol	291	370	378	359	357	294	322	288	256	218	159	158	144
Marijuana/Hashish	438	510	529	579	507	520	537	503	422	419	392	359	378
Heroin/Other Opiates	12	21	18	19	20	22	28	21	22	34	28	22	25
All Others	37	48	54	29	29	40	54	58	48	26	25	18	22
Total	778	949	979	986	913	876	941	870	748	697	604	557	569

Data Source: Vermont Substance Abuse Treatment Information System (SATIS)
This reflects only people receiving treatment at state-funded treatment facilities.

Updates can be found here: http://healthvermont.gov/adap/clearinghouse/publications.aspx#top

In addition, Medicaid recipients are receiving buprenorphine, through a prescription from a physician, to treat opioid addiction. The same individuals may also be receiving treatment within the Alcohol and Drug Abuse Programs Treatment System above.

Number of people treated with buprenorphine for Opioid Addiction in the Medicaid System by year, Vermont

Substance	2000	2001	2002	2003	2004	2005	2006	2007	2008	2009	2010	2011	2012
Heroin/Other Opiates	0	0	0	77	333	731	1107	1420	1879	2366	2693	2803	2699

Data Source: Vermont Medicaid Paid Claims
This reflects only people receiving buprenorphine to treat opioid addiction.

2. **Is there a relationship between the increased abuse of prescription opioids and the increased use of illegal opioids, such as heroin? If so, please describe that relationship.**

There is a relationship between prescription pain reliever misuse and heroin use according to the published literature. Two important resources are listed below showing direct relationships between prescription drug misuse and heroin use. The critical conclusions are included in addition to each citation.

Substance Abuse and Mental Health Services Administration (SAMHSA) Data Review[i]
- Nonmedical pain reliever users were 19 times more likely to have used heroin in the prior year
- The majority of nonmedical pain reliever users do not progress to heroin
- There is no standard path to nonmedical use of pain relievers

National Institute on Drug Abuse Fact Sheet[ii]
- Nearly half of young people who inject heroin surveyed in three recent studies reported abusing prescription opioids before starting to use heroin
- Some individuals reported taking up heroin because it is cheaper and easier to obtain than prescription opioids.
- Many of these young people also report that crushing prescription opioid pills to snort or inject the powder provided their initiation into these methods of drug administration

3. **What percentage of Vermont residents who end up addicted to opioids or heroin, or who seek treatment for such an addiction, begin their illegal drug use with, or also abuse, marijuana?**

Please note that the information listed below is based on client self-reported use. Clients may report only what he or she considers problem use, rather than any use. Alcohol use is also provided for comparison.

Vermont treatment data indicates that of those receiving treatment for opioid addiction between 2007 and 2012, 34% also indicated the use of marijuana or hashish. More than 99% of those using marijuana or hashish began using these substances prior to using opioids and typically report first use of marijuana four years before beginning to use opioids.

Of those receiving treatment for opioids between 2007 and 2012, 22% indicated also using alcohol. Nearly 96% of these individuals indicated using alcohol prior to opioids and typically report using alcohol five years before beginning to use opioids.

Please keep in mind that correlation isn't cause. Of Vermonters with marijuana as primary substance, only 14 percent also reported the use of opioids. According to the Institute of Medicine of the National Academy of Sciences:

"Patterns in progression of drug use from adolescence to adulthood are strikingly regular. Because it is the most widely used illicit drug, marijuana is predictably the first illicit drug most people encounter. Not surprisingly, most users of other illicit drugs have used marijuana first. In fact, most drug users begin with alcohol and nicotine before marijuana — usually before they are of legal age.

In the sense that marijuana use typically precedes rather than follows initiation of other illicit drug use, it is indeed a "gateway" drug. But because underage smoking and alcohol use typically precede marijuana use, marijuana is not the most common, and is rarely the first, "gateway" to illicit drug use. There is no conclusive evidence that the drug effects of marijuana are causally linked to the subsequent abuse of other illicit drugs."[iii]

4. You mentioned in your written testimony that you "see hope and progress in the 2013 Vermont Youth Risk Behavior Survey results that shows use of tobacco, alcohol, and prescription drugs by Vermont youth declined significantly from 2011 – all priorities for our community-based prevention efforts." Is reducing marijuana use among youth also part of your community-based prevention efforts to battle opioid abuse? If not, should it be? What are the trends in the use of marijuana among Vermont youth from 2011 reflected in this survey?

Reducing marijuana use among youth is a part of our community-based prevention efforts to battle opioid abuse and misuse. However more needs to be done to raise awareness about the health and safety consequences of marijuana use. Reducing the percent of high school students who use marijuana one or more times during the past 30 days is a Healthy Vermonters 2020 Goal. Those goals can be found here: http://healthvermont.gov/hv2020/dashboard/alcohol_drug.aspx. Trend data (looking at data over multiple years) has remained flat (unchanged) for past 30 day marijuana use among high school students, and has not decreased significantly since 2005 (see graph below).

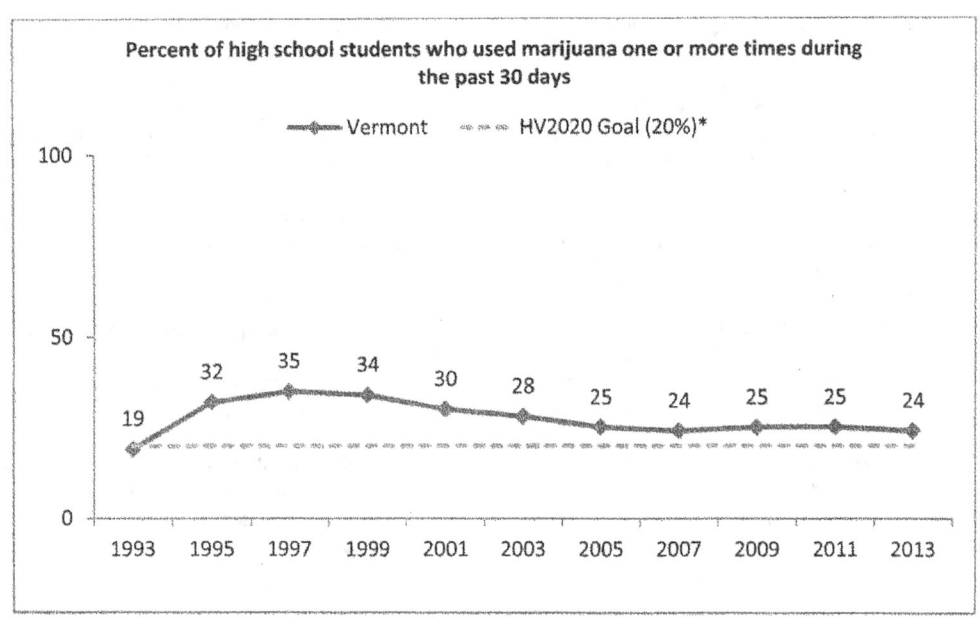

The percentage of students who think that high school students their age are at great risk of harm if they smoke marijuana **has** decreased significantly, from 34% in 2011 to 31% in 2013. Such a drop in perception of risk can lead to increased use in the future. This is of concern for our state because Vermont's marijuana prevalence rates are already higher than the national norm.

Of all high school students, 24% reported using marijuana in the past 30 days, of those, 16% also reported using a prescription pain reliever. Of all high school students, 5% reported misusing a prescription pain reliever in the past 30 days, of those 74% also reported using marijuana in the past 30 days. This is not causal – marijuana use doesn't necessarily lead to the misuse of prescription pain relievers.

We have evidence that a comprehensive prevention approach is effective. A 2012 evaluation of the Strategic Prevention Framework State Incentive Grant (SPF-SIG), funded by the Substance Abuse and Mental Health Services Administration, found those Vermont communities that augmented school and family-based prevention programs with a community education focus on marijuana collectively achieved significant reductions in marijuana use among school aged youth, as compared to other Vermont Communities. (Source: Vermont Department of Health, *SPF-SIG Project Leads to Reductions in Underage Drinking and Marijuana Use*, April 2012)

The following is a brief summary of prevention efforts headed by the Vermont Department of Health, Alcohol and Drug Abuse Programs that directly impact marijuana use.

Combined Community Prevention Grants (CCPG) are a joint initiative, supported by funding from Alcohol and Drug Abuse Prevention, Nutrition and Physical Activity, and Tobacco Control. The goal of this year's program is to support effective and integrated public health programs and communities with the capacity to respond to public health needs , and to produce healthy communities where Vermonters can lead healthy lives. Evidence-based strategies and programs that impact marijuana use that are funded by the CCPG include Community Mobilization, Media Advocacy, Screeening and Brief Intervention, Educational and Parenting Programs.

ADAP supports twenty-one supervisory unions and school districts with grants to deliver substance abuse prevention and early intervention services as part of a coordinated school health program. Evidence-based school prevention programs can save Vermont $18 for every $1 invested.[2] Examples of ADAP supported school-based services that would impact marijuana use include:

- Substance abuse screening and referral
- Coordinated school health initiatives
- Classroom health curricula
- Parenting programs
- Teacher and support staff training
- Delivery of educational support groups

Partnerships for Success (PFS) is a three-year Department of Health and Human Services, Substance Abuse and Mental Health Services Administration (SAMHSA) Grant. This project builds on the significant outcomes achieved through the Strategic Prevention Framework. Activities that would directly impact marijuana use funded under the PFS grant are parenting programs, community mobilization and media advocacy.

In addition, the state funds Project Rocking Horse, a local educational support group for low-income mothers. During the program's first year, participants increased their perception of risk from drinking or smoking during pregnancy. Those who participated in the program also gained increased confidence in the ability to handle stress and parent their children.

---

[1] **Substance Abuse and Mental Health Services Administration (SAMHSA) Data Review**
"This nationally representative study finds a strong association between prior nonmedical use of pain relievers and the subsequent past year initiation of heroin use. There are two key findings that were observed in this study. First, the recent (12 months preceding interview) heroin incidence rate was 19 times higher among those who reported prior NMPR use than among those who did not report NMPR use (0.39 vs. 0.02 percent; $0.39 \div 0.2 \cong 19$). There are many plausible explanations for this finding, including the gateway theory of drug use that posits that the use of some drugs may expose individuals to a repertoire of biological and behavioral factors that could influence their future use of other drugs. In this case, NMPR use may precondition one to engage in heroin use because prescription pain relievers have a similar pharmacological effect as that of heroin, given their similarities in chemical structure. Although the findings indicate that NMPR use is a common step on the pathway to heroin initiation, most NMPR users do not progress to heroin use. Second, heroin use appears to be neither a sufficient nor a necessary condition for the subsequent onset of NMPR use. Put differently, it appears that there are many unique pathways leading to NMPR use, and many of those do not involve heroin as a developmental precursor, or milestone, on the career trajectory of an illicit drug user."

Muhuri P, Gfroerer J, Davies M. Associations of Nonmedical Pain Reliever use and Initiation of Heroin Use in the United States. *SAMHSA CBHSQ*. 2013. http://www.samhsa.gov/data/2k13/DataReview/DR006/nonmedical-pain-reliever-use-2013.pdf

[ii] "Prescription opioid pain medications such as Oxycontin and Vicodin can have effects similar to heroin when taken in doses or in ways other than prescribed, and they are currently among the most commonly abused drugs in the United States. Research now suggests that abuse of these drugs may open the door to heroin abuse. Nearly half of young people who inject heroin surveyed in three recent studies reported abusing prescription opioids before starting to use heroin. Some individuals reported taking up heroin because it is cheaper and easier to obtain than prescription opioids. Many of these young people also report that crushing prescription opioid pills to snort or inject the powder provided their initiation into these methods of drug administration."

National Institute on Drug Abuse. U.S. Department of Health and Human Services, National Institutes of Health. http://www.drugabuse.gov/publications/drugfacts/heroin

[iii] Joy J. et. al. Marijuana and Medicine: Assessing the Science Base. Institute of Medicine. 1999 http://www.nap.edu/openbook.php?record_id=6376&page=99

RESPONSES OF MARY ALICE MCKENZIE TO QUESTIONS SUBMITTED BY SENATOR GRASSLEY

Senate Judiciary Committee

"Community Solutions to Breaking the Cycle of Heroin and Opioid Addiction"

March 17, 2014

Questions for the Record from Ranking Member Charles E. Grassley

Mary Alice McKenzie, Executive Director, Boys and Girls Club, Burlington, VT

1. *You mentioned that you have learned from youth in Burlington that there needs to be a consistent message provided to them about the dangers associated with drug use, even from an early age. As you wrote in your prepared testimony, kids have told you and your organization: "If you first start talking to me about drugs in high school, you are way too late. I smoked my first joint at (pick a number) from 8 to 12 years old."*

    Do you believe that an important part of the community's prevention efforts to battle opioid abuse should include discouraging youth from using all kinds of illegal drugs, including marijuana? How has the recent debate over legalizing marijuana affected the ability of groups like yours to transmit a consistent message along these lines?

    Senator Grassley, Thank you for asking this important question. The Boys & Girls Club in Burlington believes that Vermont should not legalize marijuana at this time.

    We believe that it is critical to do everything in our power to discourage children and youth from using all addictive substances, including marijuana, alcohol and tobacco. We believe that we must create more effective prevention programs that are sustainably funded, consistently messaged and that begin at much earlier ages. We believe that in addition to more treatment options, better funded and coordinated law enforcement, Vermont needs to create a culture of health through more effective prevention efforts regarding all addictive substances, including marijuana, alcohol and tobacco.

Senate Judiciary Committee

"Community Solutions to Breaking the Cycle of Heroin and Opioid Addiction"

March 17, 2014

Questions for the Record from Ranking Member Charles E. Grassley

<u>**Colonel Thomas L'Esperance, Director, Vermont State Police**</u>

1. In addition to heroin, what other illegal drugs are being distributed in Vermont? What do you estimate are the quantities of those other drugs being distributed and how do those quantities compare to heroin?

    The Vermont Drug Task Force (VDTF) investigates the sale and distribution of all illicit and controlled drugs. The following percentages represent the types of investigations conducted by the VDTF in 2013.

    Powder cocaine – 6%
    Crack cocaine – 22%
    Heroin – 45%
    Marijuana – 3%
    Methamphetamine - <1%
    Prescription drugs (opiate) – 17%
    Other – 6%

2. Do you believe that fully legalizing recreational marijuana, as Colorado and Washington states have done, would have a positive effect on Vermont's efforts to combat the crisis in opioid abuse?

    No. Law enforcement in Vermont devotes very little time and resources to existing marijuana laws. Legalizing marijuana could in fact have the opposite effect on law enforcement resources. Instead of freeing up resources, legalization could cause additional unforeseen crimes to increase including, but not limited to; driving under the influence of marijuana, theft and robbery from marijuana dispensaries/stores, and increases in organized crime activity related to the sale of marijuana and the cash business it generates.

MISCELLANEOUS SUBMISSIONS FOR THE RECORD

Dear Senator Leahy,

First, I would like to thank you for being an advocate for health in Vermont, particularly with regards to substance abuse prevention. Although I do work for public health, I am writing this letter solely as a citizen of Vermont and not a representative of my employer.

I am very concerned about the recent images that have portrayed Vermont as the "Heroin Capital of the US". A 14 year old friend of mine told me this weekend that Vermont has the highest rate of heroin use in the country.
This inaccurate messaging is harmful because it can socially norm the abuse of a substance if you believe "everyone is doing it".

Vermont actually ranks #41 in Heroin use (breakdown of NSDUH data in 2012). Our Youth Risk Behavior Survey just released in January also shows a decrease of heroin use and the only drugs increasing in use are marijuana and stimulants.

Heroin use in Vermont is at less than 1% (VT prevalence (2011-2012) = 0.07% while US prevalence is 0.25%)- NSDUH

While it is true our treatment rates have increased in the past decade, that is mostly due to Vermont offering better treatment options for opiate abusers (methadone and suboxone). This increase in treatment does not equate to an increase in use/abuse and this fact is getting misrepresented on many important levels.

I also think more treatment is needed for all drugs of abuse, not just opiates, and that treatment needs to be more available for all populations, particularly adolescents. Singling out opiates is like going to the bottom of the water fall instead of starting at the top and preventing people from going in the river at all.

While I agree that opiate abuse is a concern, we have the highest rates of alcohol, marijuana and cocaine use in the country and yet, we are doing little to make the connection between the use of these substances and opiates. We also are doing little to address marijuana or cocaine as a state. We cannot simultaneously be addressing the opiate issue while preparing to legalize marijuana, and not understand the connection. Early onset use of any substance contributes down the line to the opiate concerns in Vermont.

As mentioned earlier, our YRBS, BRFSS and NSDUH data all show improvement across the state in prevalence rates, yet this fact has been overshadowed since the State of the State portrayed Vermont as it did.

Vermont scored 10 out of 10 on a Robert Wood Johnson report in implementing prevention strategies for prescription drug abuse. We ranked
#1 in the country for our efforts as mentioned here:
http://healthyamericans.org/reports/drugabuse2013/release.php?stateid=VT.

I encourage members of this hearing to deeply review all the data we have in the state in order to best assess the use of limited funds to address these issues and to continue to implement research based prevention, intervention, treatment and recovery. We know what works well in prevention for example, and our numbers in Vermont show we are making a difference.

Thanks, Robin Rieske
Brattleboro, VT

My name is Nancy Corsones. I have been a trial court judge in Vermont since January of 1997. I will be unable to attend the public hearing on March 17 given my work obligations in the Bennington Criminal Division. However, I wanted to write to first thank Senator Leahy for his steadfast commitment to combatting the scourge of substance abuse and drug related crime in our community. Over a decade ago, Senator Leahy was instrumental in securing a $500,000 grant to fund Vermont's first federally funded treatment court in the Rutland Criminal Court. Together with the ongoing support of the Vermont Legislature, and many community and government partners, the Rutland County Treatment Court remains a vital resource in our community response to addiction and crime. The drug court treatment model has expanded to several other counties in our state and is now an integral part of the criminal justice system in those counties.

My request is that the drug court treatment model be fully funded, staffed and implemented in every county in Vermont. The concept of therapeutic jurisprudence in the form of treatment court has proven its value in Rutland, Chittenden, Windsor and Washington Counties over the last decade. Yet, if we don't make a treatment court model available in every county, we are running the risk of having a two tiered justice system in response to drug related crime. Those defendants who reside in a county with a treatment court have access to a far more coordinated, informed, thoughtful and successful response to their criminal conduct than do defendants who live in counties which don't have the money, staff and other resources which are vitally necessary in order to implement a successful court response to addiction driven crime. I am very concerned about the inherent disparities which result from the lack of a coordinated statewide treatment court docket.

Certainly the statewide implementation of treatment court requires substantial expenditures of money, time and staff. Many counties in our state do not currently have adequate judicial and other court resources to promptly and successfully respond to drug related crime, much less do these counties have adequate addiction treatment resources. The demand is great and we cannot underestimate the investment which will be required to successfully implement and manage treatment dockets state wide. However, the cost of implementing a treatment docket in each county must be balanced against the current staggering costs of addiction, crime and recidivism. We in Vermont have consistently proven that treatment courts are successful. Now, every part of the state must have access to the chance to successfully respond to drug related crime.

Thank you.
Nancy Corsones

QUESTION/PROPOSAL
March 10. 2014

Should it come to be the case that Rutland, VT, is selected as a federal model for dealing with opiate drug addiction it seems likely that tax dollars will flow to Vermont. Under such circumstances what kinds of work programs will be available after a person's 'graduation' from a treatment center?

Just here in Rutland there will be hundreds of x-users. Should the notion actually be to reintegrate these people into some kind of normalcy, then it seems to me because of their emotional fragility their lives will need structure, regularity, security, work, supervision, relapse treatment and an income that will afford the goal of a job, a home life, a relationship and a family.

Because these people will constitute a large potential work force I would like to make a proposal. In light of the crumbling and deteriorating water, street and sidewalk infrastructure in Rutland City that federal grant money be accessed to start a 20 year Infrastructure Works Program coordinated with the model drug program. Rutland City, like most American cities, has deferred necessary improvements for a very long time due to a lack of political will to raise taxes, and because minimum and competitive wage jobs do not result in much tax revenue and the population has decresed in Rutland. It is my contention that such a program would be a potential rational place to put people to work to get their lives together because all of the above criteria could be fulfilled. Remember, Rutland's native sons are descendents of the immigrants who came from Europe and mostly did the labor in the quarries, the marble mills, factories and railroads. PROJECT VISION seems to be in the process of establishing the treatment/corrections/mental health/social infrastructure to be effective in this role, too.

Hopelessness, disenfranchisemnt, marginalization, poverty and ignorance fracture a person's integrity. Without a reliable and liveable paycheck, relapse seems a given. For those capable of demanding physical work, grunt work to be exact, then for those persons psychologically ready such a formula of getting real pay for real work over a period of many years, overseen by the network of social service professionals in PROJECT VISION such an approach could provide an avenue through which many individuals could find meaning and a way back into life.

Since we're talking about a model national program, and because the basic national infrastructure is falling apart, it is my hope that consideration be given to creating a structure for able-bodied persons to do wholesome hard physical labor. First, here in Rutland, then nationally.

Nick Santoro

Rutland, Vermont

Comment

March 14, 2014

It is my understanding that the Vermont public school system and state correctional institutions have a hefty hand in the generation of the opioid epidemic. I never hear of this issue being addressed.

When our institutions deal with individual "deviant" behavior, by using an easy chemical fix through the use of prescription medications like Ritalin for young kids rather than with physical exercise, learning patterns, diagnostics and counseling they facilitate the sale and future use of opiates to vulnerable individuals. It is a destructive conditioning process often imposed upon young students, and DOC's conditioning upon slightly older prisoners.

Whatever programs are actively pursued to deter our opioid drug epidemic they are built on a house of cards without addressing this underlying structure that is designed by the Department of Education and/or the Department of Corrections to control people cheaply rather than addressing their needs with counseling, work programs and individualized education.

When kids leave school who are illiterate and a large proportion of our inmate population is illiterate as well drugged, and then leave prisons these people are already hooked with a predilection toward opiate drug use and other forms of drug abuse.

Nick Santoro

Rutland, Vermont

1) There are issues where doctors are over prescribing creating addiction. Why isn't there a national data base that the doctors are required to go to be for prescribing narcotic drugs? Why aren't police allowed or even a civilian to monitor the data base in Vermont for doctor shopping. Narcotic prescriptions should be limited in amount and the time period they are prescribed for. The doctors should be made accountable for over prescribing with penalties.

2) Marijuana is considered a gate way drug to other narcotic drugs, why isn't the federal government stepping in on the legalization of marijuana? I find it odd that state and federal government are allowing the legalization of marijuana for many different reasons some are as follows. The government has determined that cigarette smoking is hazardous to your health, it has been a proven fact that smoking marijuana is 2-3 times worse for you then cigarette smoking. This will be a burden cost to our health care system which the "WORKING" person will be paying for, mostly the middle income families. What's going to happen with the highway safety, workmen's compensation issue in the work place etc.

3) Will there be more funding for treatment centers throughout the New England states? Currently there are people looking for treatment and there is a delay of days, weeks and even months before they can get the treatment they need. It is crucial that treatment be available when it is needed.

4) It has been determined that whether a person receives treatment in and or out of prison basically has the same results. With this in mind treatment centers should be established in Vermont where the process allows for treatment on the outside if criminal charges for possession are charges the person has. Having weekly drug test while they are out receiving treatment to make sure that the treatment is working and they are staying off drugs. If the test come back positive, after the first or second time then they are returned to the correctional facility to finish out the time for the criminal charge and receive treatment in a secured environment.

Just a few of my thoughts on the topic.

Doug

Douglas S Johnston
Chief of Police
Springfield Police Department
201 Clinton Street
Springfield, Vermont 05156
Phone # 802-885-2113
Fax # 802-885-2235
Douglas.Johnston@state.vt.us

Dear Panel Members:

There is a greeting among some African Tribes that goes a bit like "How are the children?" Tribesmen believe that a tribes' well-being can be measured by the well-being of its children. If the children are content and thriving then the tribe will be well and all things balanced. So, rather than ask how the tribe is doing, the question becomes "How are the children?" when leaders meet.

I have lived in this community, raised my family here, and buried my parents, grandparents and great-grandparents here. When I relocated my family to Rutland I made the decision with strong conviction that it was the best place for my children. Rutland was going through a "resurrection" with so many family friendly social events and lots of new "niche" restaurants and shops downtown. We joyfully rang in the New Year with the community during First Night and hunted for bargains at the much anticipated Side Walk Sales of August.

Rutland struggled with a new element, gangs had begun to set territory here, and Los Solidos had a presence in selected neighborhoods. The children in some areas mimicked the gangs with their own naïve, imitation of a gang, FPG. Police took to the task, the public got involved and the easily identified Los Solidos seem to fade away, but they left something behind. They blazed a trail for easy trafficking of opiates and cleared the way for future dealers by creating a demand in the lower socio economic areas they discovered.

Addiction does not happen by supply alone. Addicts are created at an early age. Clinical empirical research now shows the change in the plasticity of brain and its development during early childhood as a result of trauma. Childhood trauma occurs when a child is neglected physically or emotionally. Emotional neglect can be the result of a poverty defined culture where housing and food are at risk and basic needs of the child are not met. The heightened level of the stress hormone cortisol in a developing brain actually changes the "hard wiring" of a brain. Childhood trauma has lifelong impact, creating a brain and neurological pathways that are very receptive to addiction and other mental disorders.

As a School Counselor in our public schools I have had many conversations with colleagues about the children we serve. One the trends identified is that we are now looking at third and sometimes fourth generations of poverty, neglect and addiction. These are often the families where children are in the system with DCF serving as custodians or parents who are monitored with Conditional Custody. The mission of DCF is "family reunification first". That's a wonderful ideology were it not for the fact that these families have no tools, resources or supports to do anything other than maintain the chaotic, neglectful homes that resulted in DCF intervention to begin with.

Creating a system that encourages children to be returned to situations where neglect is present does one thing very well. The system creates a future generation of addicts and strong candidates for mental illness.

Therefore, to answer how our community came to this opiate infused place we must ask ourselves the question, "How are the children?"

Respectfully,

Gina Fucci, LSC,MS

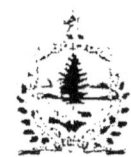

ALL LAMOILLE COUNTY
EMERGENCIES
DIAL - 911

Roger Marcoux, Jr.
Sheriff

Administration: (802) 888-3502
Civil Process: (802) 888-2561
FAX: (802) 888-2562

STATE OF VERMONT
LAMOILLE COUNTY SHERIFF'S DEPARTMENT
Post Office Box 96
Hyde Park, Vermont 05655

TESTIMONY OF SHERIFF ROGER M. MARCOUX, JR.
SENATE COMMITTEE ON THE JUDICIARY
MARCH 12, 2014

WRITTEN TESTIMONY BY
ROGER M. MARCOUX, JR.
LAMOILLE COUNTY SHERIFF
HYDE PARK, VERMONT

My name is Sheriff Roger Marcoux and I would like to thank Senator Leahy and the Senate Judiciary Committee for the opportunity to share my thoughts on the effect that opioids have on our rural communities.

I first became a police officer in 1980 and in 1984 I was assigned to the Drug Enforcement Administration Task Force (DEATF) operating from its base in Burlington, Vermont. I worked there until January 1996 when I accepted a temporary assignment with the U.S. Embassy in Port au Prince, Haiti. I was assigned to the newly formed Haitian National Police Special Investigations Unit, charged with investigating politically motivated assassinations. In February 2001 Governor Howard Dean appointed me the Sheriff of Lamoille County. I am one of the members on the Executive Board of the New England High Intensity Drug Traffic Area Program (NEHIDTA).

As background, Lamoille County is located in North Central Vermont and has a population of about 25,000. It has a total area of 464 square miles encompassing ten towns, including Stowe, which is a large ski area. As of August 2013 Lamoille County has an unemployment rate of 3.8%.

During my 12 years in the DEA Task Force at the Burlington Resident Office the overwhelming majority of our cases involved cocaine and marijuana trafficking. Between 1984 and 1996 I would be very surprised if the Burlington Resident Office submitted more than five or six heroin cases to the U.S. Attorney's Office in Vermont. The State Drug Task Force investigated several heroin cases in the Northeast Kingdom. Seldom did cases arise in Chittenden County. After being away for less than six years, I came back to find that in 2001 my own county (Lamoille) had a heroin ring in which various traffickers were traveling to Massachusetts and back with wholesale amounts of heroin, supplying the majority of the addicts in Lamoille County. The local law enforcement community and DEA worked together and arrested the local traffickers, seized their base of operations, and subsequently arrested and convicted the Massachusetts suppliers. In December 2002 the U.S. Attorney and the Attorney General of Vermont convened a conference at the State House regarding the heroin problem in Vermont. There is much documentation from the December meeting identifying the same heroin related issues that are again the focus in Vermont.

The Vermont community drove heroin underground, thus the door opened for diverted prescription drug abuse. Whether it is Vermont's cities or Vermont's rural communities, the impact of addiction is the same. Lives with potential are destroyed, families of addicts have been devastated, and in many cases these families have been nearly bankrupted attempting to save their loved ones.

According to the 2/26/14 updated Data Brief: Vermont Drug-Related Fatalities 2004-2013, "public attention has been primarily focused on prescription opioid misuse and abuse". The figures provided by the Medical Examiner's Office indicate that with all fatalities involving an opioid, the **majority** also involved multiple substances such as oxycodone, alcohol, and cocaine. Heroin is a significant public health issue in Vermont but diverted pharmaceutical drugs remain the deadliest. The Vermont Department of Health indicates that from 2004 to the end of 2013 there have been 517 deaths involving opioids, of which 456 deaths have been attributed to pharmaceutical opioids and 61 deaths to heroin. In 2013 there was a spike in heroin related deaths. Of the 94 drug related overdose deaths 50 were attributed to opioids and 21 to heroin. In 2011 and 2012 there were 18 heroin deaths combined.

The rural communities in Vermont have seen significant evidence indicating the effects of opioids. As a sheriff who provides comprehensive law enforcement services to three Lamoille towns, I have met with or heard from citizens who have been victimized either by robbery, burglary, financial crime, theft or violence. The addiction provides the motivation to commit the crime. Rural communities have smaller populations; therefore the availability of services is diminished or often non-existent. Access to treatment, prevention education, and law enforcement services is much more prevalent in the metropolitan areas of Vermont. Statewide, people with addiction have complained that there are not enough treatment facilities available. Through the years I have learned that an opportunity is often missed if treatment is not immediately available for an addict who requests assistance. By the next day that individual may no longer be interested in treatment.

 Lamoille County is in the process of establishing a Rapid Intervention for Community Change Program (RICC) based on the model initiated in Chittenden County. This program will identify repeat offenders, will focus on public health strategies providing rapid access to treatment, and will use more science based risk assessments. RICC is designed for non-violent misdemeanors. Addressing infractions rapidly is much more likely to produce results. Waiting for court dates six weeks away does not provide the same sense of urgency for the individual involved. In Lamoille County no less than 33% of the offenders entering the Lamoille County Diversion Program have admitted to being addicted to opioids.

Statewide narcotics enforcement in Vermont is comprised of the DEA Task Force and the Vermont Drug Task Force (led by Vermont State Police). Lamoille County has provided DEATF with a deputy for approximately eight years. This person is under the direct supervision of DEA. Both the DEA and VSP units are extremely busy and from my viewpoint, overwhelmed. I understand that the metropolitan areas, specifically Burlington and Rutland, are the busiest trafficking areas in the state. I also realize that we have an International border further stretching our investigative resources. As enforcement efforts become prevalent in certain areas, rural communities begin to see more out of state drug traffickers pushed into their communities. This manifests itself specifically through crimes incidental to drug trafficking, such as violence. The addiction component is driving much of the burglaries, car break-ins, and quality of life crimes.

Rural communities do not have the law enforcement resources where dedicated investigators can be assigned to disrupt drug trafficking. There are long periods of time when many communities do not receive the services from either DEATF or VSP-VDTF. This is not being critical of those agencies; it is simply a reality given their workload. I believe that it is the responsibility of every community to assist

2

those teams. Local police and sheriffs should work together regionally to know who the traffickers are within their communities. They should assist DEATF and VDTF by providing information that would expedite investigations into major drug traffickers in that local jurisdiction. DEA has a resident diversion investigator who works closely with law enforcement throughout the state. This is a relatively new position within the state but has had a significant impact. VDTF is very active and travels great distances to serve as many Vermonters as they can, but there are too few investigators.

The State of Vermont, through Governor Peter Shumlin, has put great emphasis on the failure of the current strategy. He has put great emphasis on treatment for addicts and has embraced the Chittenden County Rapid Intervention model for providing immediate attention to those in our judicial system. In addition, I would like to see an emphasis on the victims of drug abuse. Victims of crime stemming from opioid addiction need to be heard and need to receive compensation for their losses. Currently there must be an individual charged with a crime before the State's Victim Compensation Program can be accessed. Many burglaries are unsolved and victims' insurance companies are difficult to work with. It is impossible to make them feel secure again after seeing their front door broken down; however, we must give them as much support as we give to the people addicted. We must never forget that victims become involved through no choice of their own.

Prevention is a logical approach to this issue and financial support must continue to be made available to our small communities. Education through schools and community outreach will make a difference. Our best chance for success is a diminished demand for drugs.

In preparation for this testimony I contacted other law enforcement officials in rural Vermont. Sheriff Trevor Colby from Essex County advised that his small county of 6,226 people is suffering greatly from the opioid epidemic. Sheriff Colby mentioned the frustration of having people in need of long term treatment being eligible only for short term care because of limitations on their insurance. His small department does what it can to curtail drug trafficking but he needs additional deputies. Sheriff Ray Allen advised that Grand Isle County Sheriffs come across syringes on a regular basis. He advised that he needs more assistance in the investigation of drug offenses. Sheriff William Bohnyak from Orange County advised that burglaries and thefts of property are common and are a direct result of the opiate drug problem. Orange County has little to no resources to fight the opiate problem from law enforcement manpower to addiction treatment to education. Major Walter Goodell of the Vermont State Police advised that his troopers working in the rural areas of Vermont are all seeing an increase in work due to the opioid and heroin epidemic. Major Goodell echoed what other police chiefs and sheriffs have said regarding the increased pressure the issue has placed on our rural communities. He is concerned not only about his troopers but also about the lack of treatment available and the strain on other social programs.

Here are suggestions as to how the Federal Government can help:

1) Continue to support the Vermont State Police Task Force. The more funding available, the more resources that can be spread throughout the state.

2) Encourage DEA, ATF, and other federal agencies to increase their presence here in Vermont.

3) Continue to support the New England High Intensity Drug Trafficker Areas Program (NEHIDTA), which supports the Northern VT HIDTA managed through DEA.

4) Encourage the expansion of VTHIDTA. Currently focused in Chittenden County, it should be expanded to other areas such as Rutland County and the Northern Border. This would make additional funding available.

5) Support federal funding for the compensation of victims.

6) Support increased federal funding for treatment, prevention, and innovative judicial programs.

7) Support the Community Oriented Policing Program (COPS) which helps in the hiring of additional police, many of whom could help rural communities.

8) Support federal funding for the Rapid Intervention for Community Change Program (RICC). Prosecutors, law enforcement, and local Criminal Justice Centers (CJC's) all provide support for this program.

9) Encourage the continued use of the Asset Seizure Program by the U.S. Attorney's Office. If they need more resources the Justice Department should make these resources available to them.

10) Small departments rely on seized assets to continue funding drug related investigations and other community initiatives.

11) Encourage discussion among State and Federal law enforcement officials on the effectiveness of training rural law enforcement officers where they could act as force multipliers for Vermont's specialized counternarcotics investigative teams.

In conclusion, opioids and heroin in Vermont are not a new phenomenon and the state's recognition of that is evident by the December 2002 Statehouse Conference. Governor Shumlin's leadership has refocused this state's efforts to identify and implement new solutions to this ongoing public health issue. Police must remain focused on providing safe communities for our citizens and treatment is an important tool in the elimination of recidivism. However, the victims of the drug epidemic have also made it very clear to me and my fellow law enforcement colleagues that if treatment succeeds we all win. The victims have also emphasized that if treatment fails we must take the necessary measures to protect our citizens and their property; therefore, incarceration must remain an option.

The Vermont Information Center and the Office of the Medical Examiner responded to my request to identify opioid related overdose deaths by town. Since 2011 there have been 184 overdose deaths in Vermont attributed to opioids, which includes heroin. Forty-nine (49) of these deaths are of unknown origin. Of the remaining 135 deaths, 74 occurred in rural communities. That represents approximately half of the overdose deaths in the state. The same information indicates metropolitan Rutland City had 10 deaths and rural Lamoille County had 8 deaths.

I ask all State and Federal officials to remain aware of the impact that the drug epidemic is having in our rural communities. Resources must be distributed equitably.

In closing, I thank Senator Leahy for always being an advocate for law enforcement in Vermont and in the nation. I am also grateful for the opportunity to submit this testimony to the Committee and am available to answer any questions that the Committee may have.

Just recently, the Vermont Department of Public Safety announced it would be equipping Vermont State Police Troopers with Narcan as part of a program to help fight this problem. While the troopers are spread out around the state, I think there needs to be careful consideration about allowing town police departments to have the same access to this medication. The idea is great, and they will probably make a difference, but I suspect the town police departments have the potential to have more benefit. In the town of Wilmington approximately 2 months ago, my ambulance service and Wilmington PD responded to an unresponsive subject. The subject had over-dosed on Heroin and was barely breathing. The Wilmington Police officer had arrived on scene a couple minutes prior to our ambulance crew, and had he been able to administer Narcan, the patient would have been breathing a couple minutes earlier. In the end, all worked out and the patient survived, but this was a very close call. Whether the Police standards training council or someone administers a program, I think the Narcan distribution needs to be opened up to all law enforcement. I suspect you will see more instances where it would be used by those local departments initially, then just VSP.

Thank you.

Bobby
Bobby Maynard, VT EMT-I '03, NECEMS I/C, AHA CPR Instructor
Deerfield Valley Rescue, Inc. – Training Officer, Fulltime Employee
Vermont EMS District #12 Training Committee Chairperson
802-464-5557 Office
802-464-4728 Fax
802-380-3462 Cell
www.dvrescue.com

Testimony of Joseph Kraus Before the United States

Senate Committee on the Judiciary

Rutland, Vermont

March 17, 2014

My name is Joseph Kraus and I am the Chairman of Project Vision. Thank-you for the opportunity to submit written comments on behalf of Project Vision.

Project Vision is a diverse coalition of over 100 social and health service agencies and organizations, schools, colleges, business organizations, the City of Rutland, local, county, state and federal probation, parole and law enforcement agencies, faith based groups, volunteers and neighbors. We have united to address the drug related challenges facing our community with the goal of making Rutland one of the healthiest, safest and happiest communities in America.

The new Chief of Police for the City of Rutland, Vermont, James Baker, initially organized our coalition with the enthusiastic support of Mayor Christopher Louras and the Board of Aldermen. We came together based on the belief that the challenges facing our community and in particular those challenges arising from substance abuse, were not going to be resolved simply by making more arrests. More specifically, we believed that we needed to address the issues underlying substance abuse and the related criminal activity and that our efforts needed to include our broader community. We also believed that meaningful change would require a new, comprehensive and more integrated collaboration among the many agencies and organizations serving our City. To facilitate our efforts we have formed three teams, each focusing on a major area of concern. Those three areas are: treating addiction and substance abuse, reducing crime and building great neighborhoods. Our primary focus has been the City's Northwest Neighborhood, which has a number of outstanding attributes and also has more than its share of challenges.

Project Vision has two core values. The first is "Collaboration for the greater good" which affirms that our goals and objectives transcend those of any particular partner. More importantly, it reflects our belief that by working together we can accomplish more than we ever could working alone. Reflecting this value, Project Vision has no independent paid staff or support structure. Instead, we rely on the resources of our many generous partners. We are very proud of our lean and highly efficient organizational structure.

Our second value is "A renewed focus on the positive- I believe in Rutland." This value is simply a recognition of the fact that the Rutland Region is blessed with an array of wonderful attributes and is an exceptional place to live and work.

Although Project Vision has only been in existence for about a year, we have already helped to bring about some significant changes in our community. Perhaps the most significant change is the new and exciting commitment to working together to address our challenges. Our silos are starting to crumble. The best example of this is the leadership demonstrated by the Rutland City Police Department in bringing together a number of social service organizations, many of which are now co-located at the Police Department, to help address the many issues underlying criminal activity in our community. These issues include, but are not limited to mental illness, family dysfunction, poverty and substance abuse.

Recognizing the importance of this effort, Chief Baker appointed Captain Scott Tucker to serve as Executive Director of Project Vision. In this capacity Captain Tucker coordinates all the activities of the Rutland Police Department and the many social agencies now co-located in our Vision Center at the Police Department as well as the activities of our numerous partners. We believe this unprecedented level of cooperation and coordination between law enforcement and the social service agencies serving our community will bring about meaningful improvement in the lives of our citizens and more effective law enforcement. Chief Baker discusses this initiative in greater detail in his remarks.

While the initiatives of the Rutland Police Department are the most notable example of a renewed spirit of cooperation within our community, it is certainly not the only example. The City's Northwest Neighborhood currently has 21 vacant or blighted buildings, which severely affect the quality of life in the neighborhood. The Rutland Redevelopment Authority (RRA), which has historically served as Rutland City's economic development entity, is seeking a $1.25 million dollar grant to demolish, restore or replace approximately half of those vacant or blighted structures in the next four years. An undertaking of this magnitude goes well beyond the ability of the RRA alone. As such, the RRA has partnered with NeighborWorks of Western Vermont, a not for profit housing organization and the Housing Trust of Rutland County to help them complete this task. It is likely there will be other partners as well. This new and exciting partnership will permit us to accomplish so much more than we ever could working alone.

This is only the beginning. We are undertaking an extensive community building effort in the Northwest Neighborhood with a variety of initiatives. Those initiatives require the close coordination of a number of organizations including the Housing Trust of Rutland County, Neighborworks of Western Vermont, The Dream Center (created by Linda Justin and her husband Bill), which helps to mentor children and families in need, the Vermont Farmers Food Center (otherwise known as the Farmers Market), various faith based groups as well as countless volunteers and neighbors. Their goal is to make the Neighborhood strong, proud and self-directed. It is our hope that this Neighborhood becomes the last place that someone would go to sell drugs or engage in illegal activities and the first place someone would look when choosing a place to live and raise a family.

Lastly, as part of Project Vision local health and human service organizations dealing with addiction and substance abuse in the greater Rutland area have come together to determine what they can do, working in concert, to help address the challenges our community faces. These organizations, committed to the health and wellbeing of Rutland county residents have given themselves the goal of reducing addiction in Rutland County to the lowest level in the State of Vermont in the years ahead.

These organizations are working more closely than ever to develop strategies to increase awareness of, and access to, all the currently available prevention and treatment programs. They are asking themselves the hard questions- Where is access to treatment a problem? Are there gaps in existing services? Do our services overlap? How can we create a system to better support those in need based on existing resources? Project Vision has created a conversation and level of cooperation that is engaging local organizations to work together to address these critical issues in new and different ways.

We have been able to accomplish much using just the local resources available to us and we will succeed even if we have to do it all by ourselves. Our goal has always been to achieve the greatest good by more efficiently using the resources that are already available in our community. Fortunately, we have outstanding partners and they have been generous with their resources.

Although we have not devoted much effort to telling our story, almost every week some new organization or individual calls to ask what they can do to help and we have never turned anyone away. This is a testament to the many good people who call this place home. We are also fortunate that Governor Shumlin has recognized the magnitude of the opiate addiction problem here in Vermont and is supporting our efforts with enthusiasm. It is reassuring to know that we have the support of so many.

We believe that our quintessentially "Vermont" response, which blends strategies that have proven effective in other areas with creative local solutions will be successful. We are also hopeful that our model can be reproduced in other communities across our country that are facing the same challenges.

We are proud of our great City and thank-you for this opportunity to share with you our efforts to make it even better.

Thank-you.

Joe Kraus

March 17, 2014

To: The Judiciary Committee on Opioid/Heroin Addiction in Rutland, Vermont

Submitted by: Madison Akin, parent, school counselor, foster parent from Clarendon, Vermont

The heroin problem in Rutland is an infectious and insidious issue. A cure for this problem will be more than a cure for Rutland. Effectively tackling drug addiction in Rutland will create a framework for other communities to address the major factors that perpetuate drug addiction and foster the growth of unhealthy communities.

I value each perspective from this qualified panel of dedicated professionals. As a community member, school counselor in the Northwest primary school, a seasoned foster parent, a mother of an adopted child born with drug exposure and a current student in a program for mental health professionals through the Child Trauma Academy, I have a few recommendations for tackling this issue.

Investing in infant/child safety is a major element in fighting and conquering the Heroin/Opioid addiction problem in Rutland. This investment is a civil right and an economic investment that can be based on extensive neurobiological findings related to trauma, brain development and intervention.

Let's start with Civil Rights

As a seasoned mandated reporter, I have experienced the current DCF standard for investigation to be ineffective related to providing safety for children and families. I have heard some version of "if a parent is providing the basics of care; a roof, food, medical attention, then children are considered to be safe enough." I heard this recently when I reported a conversation that I had with a child who drew a picture of her mother's heroin needle for me. The child reported that the numbers that she learned in her kindergarten class were the same numbers on the needle…. "14, 15, and how do you read the next one? 16." I have watched many children show me how to crush and snort pills, smoke a bong, provide sexual favors, watch sexual favors and talk about being hungry. I know from articles in the local paper that the same parents are being arrested for drug related crimes. The children know what their parents are doing and they know not to talk about it at school.

Many of the parents are not providing any "basic level of care" because State programs are providing shelter, food, medical access and transportation. I have heard from DCF workers and parents themselves "just because a parent uses heroin does not make them unable to care for their children." I have also heard, repeatedly, "if a child reports that a parent can be woken up, than the parent is not passed out. The parent can therefore take care of the children in an emergency." The burden of the responsibility of identifying and reporting "passed out verses sleeping" levels of drug use falls on the reporting child who is usually between the ages of 5 and 8 years old. Those statements go against common sense, science and the experiences that school and mental health employees have with children from drug involved homes.

Our community is poised to provide comprehensive, best practice interventions for families who are somehow motivated to achieve a healthy home environment. We have the structure to do this through programs offered by Rutland Mental Health, Rutland Regional Medical Center and private providers. However, our judicial system is not drawing a bottom line of safety for infants and children when engagement in a variety of programs is refused. Sometimes, children need to be removed from their homes in order to avoid the horrors of Complex Trauma.

Let's move on to the Science

Taking the data and knowledge that we have from a multitude of studies, scientists and institutions and turning that into social policy requires a great deal of planning and expertise. There are a multitude of professionals from a variety of perspectives willing to work together to get the bridge between science and policy right. It can be done and there are infants born at Rutland Regional Medical Center every week who need you/us to get it right now. Their individual futures and the future of the Heroin/opioid culture of Rutland depend on you carefully imagining the weight of the following brief sound bite of the effects of being raised in a drug addicted home. (I am aware that I am speaking in generalizations about what occurs in drug addicted homes, but I am not speaking beyond the science of Trauma.)

According to the National Child Traumatic Stress Network, "the term complex trauma describes both children's exposure to multiple traumatic events, often of an invasive, interpersonal nature, and the wide-ranging, long-term impact of this exposure. These events are severe and pervasive, such as abuse or profound neglect. They usually begin early in life and can disrupt many aspects of the child's development and the very formation of a self. Since they often occur in the context of the child's relationship with a caregiver, they interfere with the child's ability to form a secure attachment bond. Many aspects of a child's healthy physical and mental development rely on this primary source of safety and stability."

My work experience in Rutland has shown me that children with drug addicted primary care providers are living in environments that expose them to situations creating Complex Trauma. The children whom I know from these environments have unhealthy home lives with degrees of domestic violence, unsafe care providers, hunger, housing instability, poverty of opportunity, neglect, and often, exposure to sexual information or direct sexual abuse.

Dr. Bruce Perry from the Child Trauma Academy, writes extensively about brain development from conception through a lifetime. Neuroscience informs that our brains develop from the most basic and primitive functions to the more complex functions of abstract thought. The first three years of our lives are disproportionately more active regarding neural pathway development and connectivity as compared to other developmental stages. According to Dr. Perry, 80% of our brains are neurologically developed by the time we are old enough for kindergarten.

This 80% of growth occurs according to the events of our lives. If those events are constant insults like irregular feedings, unresponsive or abusively responsive primary care interactions, fear, and discomfort, our brains will orient towards trauma development. A child in that environment will have a different resting heart rate, different arousal patterns, and different gastro intestinal makeup, when compared to a healthy child. Left in that environment, a child's brain will develop neural networks that will make being an emotionally stable, emotionally regulated adult extremely challenging.

According to Bessel van der Kolk, MD, Complex Trauma creates seven domains of impairment for exposed children. Children who develop in hostile or neglectful environments must then manage the results of a trauma altered brain. The following domains highlight some of the challenges that will persist, in some compacity, over a lifetime and create challenges for individuals and therefore society.

1) Attachment (ie: problems with boundaries, social isolation, interpersonal difficulties, attuning difficulty)

2) Biology (ie: sensorimotor development problems, problems with coordination, balance and body tone)

3) Affect regulation (ie: difficulty with emotional self-regulation, difficulty labeling and expressing feelings, problems knowing and describing internal states, difficulty communicating wishes and needs)

4) Dissociation (ie: distinct alterations in states of consciousness, impaired memory for state-based events, two or more distinct states of consciousness)

5) Behavioral control (ie: poor modulation of impulses, self-destructive behavior, aggression toward others, pathological self-soothing behaviors, sleep disturbances, eating disorders, substance abuse, excessive compliance, oppositional behavior, difficulty complying with rules, reenactment of trauma in behavior or play

6) Cognition (ie: difficulties in attention regulation and executive functioning, lack of sustained curiosity, problems with focusing on and completing tasks, problems understanding responsibility, learning difficulties, problems with language development)

7) Self –concept (ie: lack of a continuous, predictable sense of self, low self-esteem, shame and guilt)

Using this information, it becomes clear that leaving children in abusive, neglectful environments for the sake of "maintaining families" is not serving the child, parent, family, community or future for anyone. If a parent is unable or unwilling to participate in therapeutic change, then the system needs to step in on the child's behalf and provide an opportunity for safety and healthy development. The current science of Trauma should support a guideline for types of intervention. If a parent refuses or is unwilling to provide basic healthy environment for a child, the judicial system, with the support of community partnerships needs to take action on the child's behalf. The action can be focused on urgent needs of the child due to age, development and danger.

The Economics of Intervention

In the fall of 2013, Assistant Superintendent of Rutland City Public Schools, Mr. Robert Bliss presented at a community forum about the financial impact that drugs are having on public schools. It would take an economist and a panel of community specialists to generate an actual dollar amount for the cost of providing a fair and equal education for a student of Complex Trauma or a student being raised in a drug involved home.

Art Rolnick, an economist from Minnesota, presented on TEDx Talks on August 8, 2011 about the economic benefit to fully funding early childhood development programs for students, especially high risk toddlers. He makes an excellent case regarding the annual rate of return that is afforded to communities who protect their young children. He initially began his work believing in the financial benefit of promoting preschool programs for the financial benefit of communities. After becoming connected with Dr. Perry and Dr. Shonkoff (co-author of the book Neurons to Neighborhoods) and understanding basic brain development, he began to talk about "early intervention" meaning prenatal to five years old.

Mr. Rolnick discussed the annual rate of return for protecting children. His formula was easy to follow and he concluded a conservative annual rate of return for protection of at risk kids (what he calls High Return Kids) at 18%. His formula included the savings for providing early interventions related to a decrease in the cost of schooling, drop in crime, improved productivity in adult life, etc. His policy and program ideas for investment in children and families have been sought after nationally with programs and research projects currently fully funded.

Let's talk about Rutland

It is challenging work to put neuroscience into social policy, but we know enough about brain development, abuse and drug addicted parents in this community to know that we are not keeping our children safe enough. We know enough about Rutland's drug problem to conclude that the current practice of "maintaining families at all costs" is not working for babies, siblings, parents, communities, the economy, school systems, peers or the criminal justice system. This policy is an attempt to respect the sanctity of the family but children and the future fabric of our society are paying the current price and will pay an emotional and financial price with each generation.

We are inadvertently providing a self sustaining environment for drug dealers and addicts by allowing addicted and using parents, who refuse to participate in treatment options, to maintain custody of their children for our interest in maintaining "family connections." In our attempt to provide moral public policy we are facilitating a policy that disregards the neurobiological data we have about children, safety and healthy development.

Intervention for our community needs to be timely, effective, strength based and supported by the current science and data that has been available for over ten years. As a community, we have the knowledge, professionals and systems to intervene on behalf of all individuals affected by Heroin and Opioid abuse. It is time to make policy changes to support the safety, health and well being of the entire community.

BPS HEALTH, LLC   56 Old Farm Rd. #2   Stowe, VT. 05672
Dr. Rick Barnett, Psy.D., LADC   Ph. 802-373-2909   Fax. 888-923-3476
Licensed Psychologist-Doctorate   NPI 1205844883   VT License #860
Licensed Alcohol and Drug Counselor

March 17, 2014

Senate Judiciary Committee
Field Hearing
Rutland, VT

Re: Community Solutions To Breaking The Cycle Of Heroin And Opioid Addiction

To The Senate Judiciary Committee:

Thank you for allowing the submission of testimony on programs and services for the
treatment of opioid abuse, which is an escalating public health crisis and an issue of major
concern to many Vermonters. As heroin and opioid addiction has become a growing and
devastating trend in Vermont as well as nationally, there has also been a massive trend in
the adoption of Medication-Assisted Treatment (MAT), with an emphasis on using
Methadone or Buprenorphine as a first-line treatment approach.

Treatment using Buprenorphine has saved many lives. It must, however, remain a tool in
the larger toolbox in the treatment of opioid addiction. Buprenorphine should be used
judiciously in conjunction with a broad-based treatment program and not as a stand-alone
treatment by a medical provider. This is because Buprenorphine is not a "safe" option: it
has been associated with an increasing number of fatalities, emergency department
episodes, and pediatric exposures. It is the drug-of-choice in prisons. It is a popular street
drug for its anti-withdrawal properties, mild euphoric effects and ease of obtaining and
selling. Considering these facts (CESAR FAX Buprenorphine Series 2/4/13):

1. Emergency Department visits for Buprenorphine increases 10-fold from 2005 to
    2010
2. 61% of Buprenorphine-Related Emergency Department visits are for non-medical
    use
3. Nearly All Emergency Department Visits for the Accidental Ingestion of
    Buprenorphine Occur in Children Under the Age of Six
4. Continuing Medical Education Improves Buprenorphine Waivered Physicians'
    Knowledge and Practice Behaviors
5. Northeastern and Southern Regions of Country Account for Largest Increases in
    Buprenorphine Found in Law Enforcement Drug Seizures
6. One-Third of U.S. Treatment Applicants Report Buprenorphine/Naloxone Sold on
    Street; One Fifth Report the Drug Is Used to Get High
    (Source: http://www.cesar.umd.edu/cesar/pubs/BuprenorphineCESARFAX.pdf)

Physicians are overwhelmed by the demand and complexities involved in treating
addictions. Decreasing numbers are accepting new patients and fewer are signing up to
obtain the 8-hour training required to prescribe the drug. [why? is this because they are
afraid of prescribing Buprenorphine?] Physicians are not addiction treatment providers

BPS HEALTH, LLC   56 Old Farm Rd. #2   Stowe, VT. 05672
Dr. Rick Barnett, Psy.D., LADC   Ph. 802-373-2909   Fax. 888-923-3476
Licensed Psychologist-Doctorate   NPI 1205844883   VT License #860
Licensed Alcohol and Drug Counselor

and MAT is not the only choice for patients struggling with opioid addiction. Health care providers and agencies, policymakers, the general public, and those struggling with addiction must move beyond the confines of "Harm-Reduction" vs. "Abstinence-Based" models of treatment for opioid addiction.

A more effective solution to opioid addiction may be investing resources in comprehensive addiction training for all health care providers, especially nurses and physicians, _and_ comprehensive treatment programs that treat all facets of addiction, not simply the physical side of addiction. Research shows that health care providers with more training on addiction may provide treatment that results in increased patient-satisfaction, decreased provider burn-out, and possibly better outcomes. Furthermore, there is ample research that shows that the combination of pharmacotherapy and psychosocial treatment consistently results in better outcomes that medication alone.

One way to change the way we discuss and treat opioid addiction is to eliminate the term "Medication-Assisted Treatment" (MAT) and replace it with the term "Counseling-Assisted Pharmacotherapy" (CAP). This simple change would re-orient patients, providers, and the public towards a more complete approach to the treatment of opioid addiction.

Another way to ensure that appropriate services and treatment are provided to those struggling with opioid addiction, thereby improving outcomes, is to integrate alcohol and substance use disorder treatments into the overall healthcare reform and redesign process. Clinical providers of substance abuse services and mental health providers need to be better aligned with and included in primary care service delivery models. For example, the current waitlist at many mental health agencies in addition to the failure to aggressively reach out to the independent mental health and substance abuse provider community demonstrates the poor organization and fragmentation of the current system.

Addiction treatment professionals, mental health providers, medical providers, and peer recovery support systems equally share in the responsibility for the treatment of and recovery from opioid addiction. Emphasizing one approach over another will result in poor outcomes. Vermont's current "Hub and Spoke" model is promising yet it continues to overvalue the "Hub", or Buprenorphine prescribing, and devalue the "Spoke", or Mental Health/Substance Abuse treatment providers. This initiative will result in better outcomes if as much emphasis was placed on the psycho-social aspect of treatment as is placed on the physical side of addiction treatment.

Respectfully Submitted,

Rick Barnett, Psy.D., LADC

BPS HEALTH, LLC   56 Old Farm Rd. #2   Stowe, VT. 05672
Dr. Rick Barnett, Psy.D., LADC   Ph. 802-373-2909   Fax. 888-923-3476
Licensed Psychologist-Doctorate   NPI 1205844883   VT License #860
Licensed Alcohol and Drug Counselor

Dr. Barnett is an alcoholic and addict in recovery for over 20 years and has worked in the field of addiction treatment and recovery and mental health services for nearly 20 years with extensive experience in hospital-based settings, residential settings, community settings, and outpatient independent practice settings. He has a Doctorate in clinical psychology, a Master's in clinical psychopharmacology, and a license in alcohol and drug counseling. His doctoral dissertation was on the education and training of physicians on alcohol and substance use disorders.

Dustin A. Degree
St. Albans, Vermont

March 17th, 2014

Mr. Chairman, Ranking Member Grassley and Members of the Judiciary Committee:

First, I'd like to thank Chairman Leahy for taking the time to continue this important national conversation here in our home state of Vermont. The level of attention opiate addiction has received -- both here and across the country -- in the last several months is a welcome sign to those of us who understand the dire consequences of continued inaction.

In some ways, Vermont has taken the lead in the search for solutions. Unfortunately, there is a direct correlation between that leadership, and the desperate need for it here in the Green Mountains. Unlike any other state, Vermont -- specifically the northwestern corner -- has been cast as the national example for the need to better understand and act to reduce opioid abuse. This hearing and others like it give us the opportunity to share the countless statistics that show the depth and breadth of this problem. It is important data that offers a variety of perspectives and builds a growing understanding of the devastating effects of this particular addiction.

However, while this may be the favored approach of government, this is a problem which will never be solved by numbers. Because each of these numbers is attached to a name. Names with faces, families and friends. I grew up with them. I went to elementary and high school with them. I watched them go off to college, become adults, start careers and families and then, one by one, watched them lose everything.

I graduated from Bellows Free Academy in St. Albans in 2003. I remember vividly when the recreational use of prescription drugs became a part of social culture. I remember the first time I saw a friend chase a generic Percocet with a beer at a party. I remember the first time I heard a classmate was using needles and heroin and I remember the first time I learned someone I knew had overdosed and died.

For the past twelve years I've watched my community change in ways that I fear may take decades to reverse. We've seen a steady rise in burglary, petty theft and other property crimes as desperation envelopes the addicted in service to a habit that has turned good kids into criminals, neighbors into victims and neighborhoods into targets. In my hometown and many others across the state, opioid abuse has drastically changed the way we live.

When I was elected to the Vermont House of Representatives from St. Albans City, I tried to convince those in power that prescription drug abuse was the single greatest problem facing my generation of Vermonters; that if left unattended it threatened to change the very character of our state.

Some understood, but too many clung to an antiquated stereotype of habitual drug use and users, a flawed perception that this problem is unique to a certain demographic of Vermonters predetermined to addiction: the poor or undereducated or those who may lack a positive support system at home. However, we know today that this problem is not socioeconomic. It's not racial or regional. It's universal.

Even now, there are some who – still – have yet to grasp the vast scope of the problem. We saw it when Governor Peter Shumlin devoted his entire State of the State Address to it, leaving some legislators and pundits on both sides perplexed as to why he would do such a thing.

Opioid abuse worth isn't a single speech. It's worth 251, given in every community to call on the people of our state to begin immediately taking steps toward a resolution.

We must find a way to ensure that anyone who seeks treatment has the appropriate resources for recovery.

We must find ways to identify and treat those addicts currently in, or entering, the criminal justice system. Not doing so is an absolute failure of the state and federal correction systems. Both of which must reemphasize rehabilitation in order reduce recidivism.

We must find better ways for federal, state, county and municipal law enforcement agencies to work together to enforce stricter penalties for diversion and sales.

And we need to build a network of drug take back centers, to reduce the amount of unused opioids, which might otherwise end up diverted and abused.

Finally, we need to remember there is no quick fix and that recovery is a lifelong battle. Our best efforts today must be matched tomorrow, and the day after. Our support must be perpetual. My generation will forever be tasked with ensuring that the path to recovery, and the support government can give to it, is an available reality for all who seek it.

Mr. Chairman, the fate of so many lies in the work done by this committee, and all others endeavored in public service, to find solutions today that will bring light to the darkness opioid addiction has cast upon too many Vermonters.

I readily join in that work with faith and confidence that this, the great battle of my generation, can be won.

My faith lives in the momentum that events just this build toward developing national policies that will move us closer to a solution. It lives in the actions of those who have fought through recovery and emerged to tell their story and share their experience in hopes of helping others reclaim freedom from addiction. And it lives in knowing that Vermonters stand willing and eager to fight for a system that ensures better outcomes for those who need help and safer communities for all of us.

Mr. Chairman, on behalf of my generation, I urge you to act.

Respectfully submitted,

Dustin A. Degree

Senator Leahy,

Good afternoon.

Today I listened to a portion of the testimony in Rutland regarding concerns about drug problems and intervention. I thank you for coming to Rutland and listening to the many speakers. Giving Rutland a voice in this is vital to our continued efforts.

What struck me was that we seem to talk around many of the underlying issues that relate to strengthening families. I work with children in an after-school tutoring program and have seen the results of families who are in themselves dysfunctional or incapable of solving very serious problems facing their children. This involves economic, health, social and emotional factors that decrease the success of family.

A recent conversation with our Assistant Superintendent of schools I think hit upon a significant need. We need to bring parents together to talk about and develop strategies so they can deal with problems facing them and their children. Parents often ask me how to deal with unruly children, or children whose significant learning challenges are not being met or children who are bullied. When children do not feel safe or do not feel supported at home they become weakened. These problems of the family may well be the elements that provide access for those individuals seeking vulnerability in our community. If parents are not at the forefront of any prevention program we cannot hope to turn around what is happening in our communities.

All of the efforts being promoted by the police, by drug rehab and prevention programs and by programs like the Boys and Girls Clubs are wonderful, but they cannot fill the void that is created when families are falling apart or not functioning well.

Thank you for listening. I hope that my comments may add to the already very thoughtful testimony given today. I was unable to attend the meeting because of my commitment to serving children, but I continue to support my city and its efforts through Project Vision.

Respectfully submitted,

Dr. Alis Headlam, Ed.D.
One World Consulting, Inc.
Tutoring that Makes Sense

I am wondering if there is any way we can down grade Ibogaine from a class 1 narcotic so it can be used in breaking the cycle of heroin addiction. Ibogaine seems to be a great idea and with regulation and affordability, we could reduce the amount of heroin and meth addicts in the US. I am a foster parent right here in Rutland County and see first hand, with my kids, how terrible this addiction is. I will do my best to be at the hearing on Monday at the Howe Center. Please address the subject of Ibogaine during the hearing. I am very happy that we have such a wonderful clinic right here in Rutland; but would be even more proud if we broke the cycle of addiction with Ibogaine.

Monica Rugg
Foster Parent and Full Time Student
Wallingford, VT

I am a Registered Nurse in a busy mother-baby unit in Vermont Many people don't realize that in addition to taking care of healthy postpartum mothers and babies, we also take care of high-risk antepartum patients. This includes opiate-addicted women in all stages of pregnancy. We are extremely fortunate to have the resources and programs in place to help these women and their babies, and I feel that we are doing right to make their treatment a priority. But I am filled with unease with the lack of treatment options for the general population and what this means for the real options opiate-addicted women feel they have.

If an addict decides that today is the day that she is ready to get help, that window is a critical one and is only open for a short time. There are significant waiting periods for treatment for opiate addiction in Vermont. But if a woman is pregnant, she gets bumped to the top of the list. Based on what I see, I worry that women sometimes get pregnant as a means to get into treatment, not because they want - or can provide for - a child. Recently, professionals from 3 major hospitals in Vermont stated that between 6 and 8% of babies born in Vermont suffer from neonatal abstinence syndrome.

It seems obvious to say that we need more treatment options and earlier interventions, but I'm going to say it here anyway. We need more treatment options, and earlier interventions! Please take this into consideration as you navigate this complex issue with our community leaders. Many thanks for your hard work!

Sincerely,
Chelsea Clark, RN, CLC
Fairfax, VT

PETER SHUMLIN
Governor

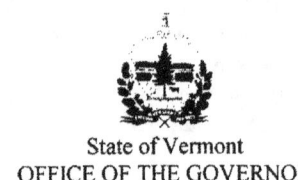

State of Vermont
OFFICE OF THE GOVERNOR

Written Testimony of Vermont Gov. Peter Shumlin

Senate Judiciary Committee Field Hearing

March 17, 2014

Rutland, Vermont

I would like to thank Chairman Leahy, Ranking Member Grassley, and other distinguished Members of the Judiciary Committee for this opportunity to provide testimony on the growing opiate and heroin crisis facing Vermont and the nation, and the work Vermont is doing right now to meet this challenge.

Vermont's economy is rebounding from the worst national recession since the depression. Our unemployment rate is among the lowest in the nation, companies are expanding, and home values are on the rise. Vermont is one of the safest states in the country, leads the nation in high school graduation rates, consistently ranks among the top states for health, exercise, and other measures of well-being, and is poised to expand our already-admirable early childhood education programs statewide.

We are also a state where neighbors know each other and care for each other. We are proud of our work ethic, our commitment to strong local communities, and the remarkable quality of life that draws employers, new residents, and visitors alike.

But Vermont is not immune to the challenges facing other states. In my judgment, the greatest threat to Vermont's strong future is the rising tide of drug addiction and related crime that is being felt here and nationally.

Across this country, heroin use rose 79 percent from 2007 to 2012, with 81 percent of first-time heroin users moving from abusing prescription drugs. Heroin overdoses claim more than 3,000 lives annually across this country, a number that is climbing. In Vermont, we have seen a nearly 260% increase in people receiving heroin treatment since 2000, nearly 40% in just the past year. There have been twice as many federal indictments against heroin dealers here in 2013 than in the prior two years, and nearly double the deaths from heroin and opioids last year as we had in the entire preceding year.

For those reasons, I chose to devote my annual State of the State address to not just acknowledging the threat, but more importantly outlining my own proposals for preventing and treating addiction, toughening laws to keep big-time dealers out of Vermont, and ensuring our families are healthy and our communities safer.

In short, I say to you today that law enforcement alone cannot stem this dangerous tide. Until we acknowledge that addiction is an illness, no different than heart disease or diabetes, we will never reverse those damaging and deadly statistics.

Today you will hear from others who are on the front lines of this battle, and I appreciate your attention to their ideas for tackling this crisis. For too long we have nibbled around the edges of this problem, rather than pursuing a comprehensive plan for moving forward.

I called for expanding staffing and space at backlogged treatment centers to ensure every addict has access to help stay clean; increasing programs through use of state and federal funding for substance abuse and mental health treatment services for Reach Up recipients; programs to keep more addicts in treatment and out of expensive jail cells where appropriate; high-quality early education programs to help young Vermonters get the best start on life possible, avoiding the pitfalls of addiction; tougher sentencing for big-time drug dealers to send a clear message that Vermont is not open for business; and much more.

We know this makes sense both morally and economically. In fact, a jail cell costs taxpayers more than $1,000 weekly, while out-patient treatment costs $136. Spending money on early education so that kids get a strong start and avoid the hopelessness and lack of opportunity that often leads to addiction will help reduce money spent putting lives back together after addiction has taken hold. I believe Vermont's comprehensive approach, which involves the treatment and medical community, judiciary, law enforcement, schools, community groups, and many others, should serve as a national model. I continue to believe that the best prevention is a great education, solid jobs, a thriving economy, and a good quality of life.

Vermont State Police Director Col. Thomas L'Esperance will testify to the vital role law enforcement plays in this effort, and I join the Colonel in thanking Sen. Leahy for helping secure the funding needed for our effective Drug Task Force. Vermont Health Commissioner Dr. Harry Chen will testify to the crucial need for prevention and treatment. Your committee is in Rutland today because of the remarkable progress members of this community, working together, have made in driving out drug crime and ensuring treatment and compassion are available for their neighbors who suffer from the disease of addiction.

Vermonters are every level are involved in the battle against addiction and the problems it brings into our homes, workplaces and communities. I want to thank all of those here today and elsewhere in Vermont who are working with those of us at the state and federal level who are committed to getting this right for Vermont.

I especially want to thank Sen. Leahy for bringing the Judiciary Committee to his home state today Acknowledging this problem and talking about it candidly is critical. For too long the stigma and shame of addiction has stifled our discussions and therefore any real progress. I also appreciate the recognition that, just as Rutland has taken a unique, community-based path to preserve its quality of life, Vermont's comprehensive approach to battling addiction can serve as a model for neighborhoods, cities and states – urban and rural – across the nation.

Thank you for your time.

I am a substance abuse counselor in Addison county. I have been in the addictions field for the past 15 years. I have a master's degree in counseling psychology and am a licensed alcohol and drug counselor. One of my biggest hurdles is the fact that the state of Vermont continues NOT to recognize my license and reimburse me for clients who have Medicaid and Medicare health insurances. Most major medical insurances recognize and reimburse the counseling work I do with clients struggling with substance abuse issues yet I have to turn away many clients who cannot afford to pay out of pocket because they have Medicaid or Medicare. When will the state of Vermont wake up and change this policy? They talk about reform and support yet they require a client to be assessed and counseled by a licensed drug and alcohol counselor but won't back their services financially. People are asking for help but are being placed on waiting lists when this simple change could help many access the services they need.

Terri Mayer Thomsen, MA, LADC

Senator Leahy,

Thank you for organizing the important hearing on drug use in Rutland. I am an Assistant Professor of Sociology at Middlebury College and a Rutland resident.

One key piece of this complicated puzzle was missing from yesterday's discussion: harm reduction. As you know, strategies that keep drug users safe are also a key to connecting them to much-needed social services, including drug treatment and housing. Syringe exchange, widely considered a vital and evidence-based public health practice that addresses the health of drug users, was not discussed at the meeting. Rutland's Chief of Police does not support syringe exchange despite its proven effectiveness at (1) reducing the harms of drug use and (2) linking people to necessary treatment.

Any effective solution to addiction must take into account the humanity of drug users. Harm reduction is one such strategy. Drug users are not "them" - they are "us". They are part of the community of Rutland. Their perspectives must be part of the solution too. I hope that you consider drug users as people deserving of harm reduction services and will emphasize this important tool as a way address the health and social services needs of drug users in Vermont.

Take Care,
Rebecca

Rebecca Tiger
Sociology/Anthropology
Middlebury College
rtiger@middlebury.edu
Author of Judging Addicts<http://nyupress.org/books/book-details.aspx?bookid=6817>

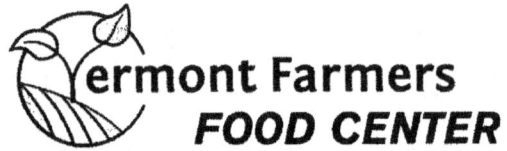 **ermont Farmers FOOD CENTER**

P.O. Box 1008, Rutland, VT 05701

www.VermontFarmersFoodCenter.org

March 18, 2014

US Senate Judiciary Committee

Senator Patrick Leahy, Chairman

Testimony on "Community Solutions to Breaking the Cycle of Heroin and Opioid Addiction

In the notorious North West neighborhood of Rutland City, a formerly derelict industrial building, now renovated and light-filled, is the Vermont Farmers Food Center (VFFC) hosting Rutland's vibrant winter farmers market, a bustling gathering place for the community to shop and socialize each Saturday. The next strategic step for VFFC in collaboration with Project Vision , involves establishing a flourishing community garden for the adjacent distressed and disinvested historic Northwest neighborhood's use at the strategic point where a great deal of pedestrian traffic from there occurs.

The raised beds will serve the dual purpose of a demonstration garden and a place where those in need of fresh, healthy produce can pick what they can use while helping to tend the gardens. The design promises it to be "a neighborhood treasure, both functional and beautiful," drawing all age groups outdoors to seed and sprout hope in their lives becoming more than they've been, gradually building their confidence to actively work together making and protecting improvements to their immediate environments while forming closer ties among themselves and more widely in the community to build personal, family and neighborhood resilience. The VFFC site will also serve as an agricultural events center with education and training the hallmark of the VFFC activities to include job training for a range of food-related occupations. Eventually, we have a kitchen on VFFC site, with food demonstrations and cooking classes featured regularly to enable more local families to learn to prepare and love healthy foods that are available in the greater Rutland area.

A Community Gardens Build Day scheduled April 12th, 2014 will be a pivotal event for the entire Rutland community, the most visually prominent step in partnership with Project VISION towards fostering community cohesiveness and stability for those most at-risk. VISION is a coalition of many local agencies, organizations, professionals and volunteers making progress in addressing a multitude of social and policing issues, the goal of which is to give Northwest residents the resources and capacity they need to create the change they seek. From volunteers joining in, VFFC will build a Peer-to-Peer Urban Farming Trainer program to provide comprehensive leadership and mentoring throughout future growing seasons. We are hoping to recruit marginalized parents needing to complete community service using this garden as an activity with their children to fill their community service requirement. What better way to heal, coming together in community, enjoying the outdoors with your kids and learning to have a relationship with the earth. Please help us with this vision. Thank you.

Kathleen Krevetski RN , VFFC

Our family has been impacted with the disease of addiction. My daughter started using Opioids 4 years ago while at college.

Now after 3 tries at rehab and now on another path of recovery with her infant son. My / our story is not uncommon.

At a time when my daughter was seeking help for herself, treatment facilities here in Vermont were offering long wait times unless the addict had a criminal record or being suicidal. This was discouraging and frustrating to her. Knowing that a criminal offense was potential, she sought treatment. To gain entrance into treatment, mentioning the thoughts of suicide gave her access to treatment.

Every addict has a different bottom that will lead them to seek help. Her story is not uncommon. Once in treatment she was able to convince herself and others that an early release was going to work for her. Relapsing is heart breaking but a known fact of addiction. Caring for her infant son and being newly into another recovery are two challenges that she and many other young women are faced with. They need to have positive people and places to turn.

In future discussions I would like to hear the thoughts on, quality aftercare opportunities and mandatory length of stay programs. Recovery / sober homes for women are very difficult to find in Vermont. Getting an addict into treatment is a start but keeping them healthy is very important.

I live in the Rutland area and find it discouraging that Rutland is being labeled as the "heroin capital of Vermont ". These are our families and our kids that are being affected by the disease of addiction. Finding solutions and trying to remove the shame lets Rutland rise above the criticism. We need to be brave enough to say we have problems lets work on this and keep moving towards positive outcomes. A community that offers opportunities to addicts that will seek help for themselves, maybe even before law enforcement is demanded. Supporting the efforts of recovery with quality aftercare gives hope of a better life here in Rutland.

In my work with women I want to state that it very often seems underlying depression/anxiety is a factor in opioid abuse. Increasing mental health care, depression screening, shortening waits for counseling and support would go a long way I think.

Another issue is of course the over prescription of potent painkillers by medical and dental providers. Too many pills being dispensed. Maybe a person needs 4-6 percocet after dental extractions. Why then prescribe 12-15? If a patient needs more, a call to office for refill could be made, also for a small amount. If you look at the history of addiction in the US, the medical community has played a part for sure. And pharmaceutical industry too.

Also, why do I see women getting opioids prescribed after a vaginal delivery when ibuprofen and Tylenol should do the trick? Recipe for trouble...

Also, why cannot pharmacies accept unwanted medication all the time, not just on those special take back days? Seems like a good way to get it out of peoples medicine cabinets before youngsters get a hold of them...

Thanks for asking, glad there was a hearing.

Jessica Doos, RN

Statement by Robert F. Forman, Ph.D.
Director, Professional Relations & Policy[1]
Alkermes, Inc.
Waltham, Massachusetts
March 17, 2014

Facing the Problem of Heroin and Opioid Addiction

Thank you, Chairman Leahy, for holding this important hearing and helping to bring attention to how communities can *Break the Cycle of Heroin and Opioid Addiction.* Likewise, we are grateful to Governor Shumlin for devoting his recent State of the State Address to this topic.

I am offering this testimony because our company, Alkermes, Inc., manufactures and markets an important, yet under-utilized medication that is approved by the U.S. Food and Drug Administration (FDA) for the treatment of opioid dependence. In the testimony that follows, I advocate for a comprehensive approach that includes the latest evidence-based treatments to address the problem of heroin and prescription opioid addiction. In addition, a multi-state project is proposed, to make opioid dependence medications and counseling available to those communities that are being most severely affected by the heroin and prescription opioid epidemic.

Addiction to heroin and prescription opioids has become one of the most challenging public health issues of our time, impacting our communities in ways that are far worse than anyone might have imagined. Opioid addiction takes young, promising lives and destroys them without regard to sex, race, religion, economic status, or any other social factor. Death may come suddenly through an overdose, or slowly, as an individual's entire life is consumed. These addictions are incredibly difficult problems for their families, too. Addictions are highly stigmatized and as such, people may prefer to simply ignore it, or minimize the extent of the problem. This is true of the addicted individual, communities and the pharmaceutical industry as well. Alkermes is one of the few companies applying modern science and advanced technologies to address the public health problem of addiction.

The situation in Vermont mirrors what is happening in many other parts of the country. In 2012, the Centers for Disease Control declared that our country was in the midst of a prescription opioid overdose epidemic[2] and, more recently, researchers have documented that the prescription opioid epidemic has now grown into an even worse problem,[3] with the dramatic return of heroin to unsuspecting neighborhoods across the country.[4]

The facts outlined in Governor Shumlin's State of the State Address plainly present the realities in Vermont:
- Treatment admissions for opioid dependence increased over 700% in the past decade;
- Admissions for treatment of heroin dependence have more than doubled in the past year.[5]

Heroin and other opioids also have a profound impact on crime. Again, Governor Shumlin's address is instructive: in 2013, there were twice as many federal indictments against heroin dealers in Vermont than in the prior two years, and more than five times as many as had been obtained in 2010.[6]

Vermont is not alone in having to face these problems. In rural and urban centers across the country, heroin use, opioid addiction, deadly overdoses and heroin-fueled crime have increased at alarming rates. A few examples from that same NIDA report confirms this point:[7]

- The Chicago metropolitan area witnessed nearly a 900% increase in overdose deaths due to heroin since 1999 - with nearly half of these deaths involving people under the age of 25;

- The Minneapolis/St. Paul area reported that heroin-involved emergency room visits nearly tripled from 2004 to 2011; and

- The Cincinnati metropolitan area county coroner's office reported a 342% increase in heroin overdose deaths since 2008.

Regrettably, we could easily add many more cities and states to this list. In fact, in the most recent NIDA study of drug trends, the return of heroin was the most cited problem.[8]

Heroin and other opioids also have a devastating impact on unborn and newborn children. In America, during every hour of every day, at least one baby is born dependent upon heroin or other opioids and in need of intensive emergency management of their physical withdrawal from opioids. In 2009, it was estimated that over 13,000 newborns underwent opioid withdrawal,[9] and more recent reports from a number of states indicate that the prevalence of *neonatal abstinence syndrome* is worsening steadily.[10]

Given the seriousness of the problem, what should we do?

Fortunately, research has led to the development of important options for treating heroin and other opioid addictions. The challenge before us is how to bring all of these evidence-based approaches to scale, not in just in a few communities, but to all of those communities that have been affected by this epidemic. We know that opioid addiction is a disease and as such, we must treat it like the public health emergency it is. We have confronted and successfully tackled other public health crises in this country. We can also confront the heroin and prescription opioid epidemic by employing a comprehensive approach that utilizes all of the evidence-based tools available to us today.

A comprehensive approach to the heroin and opioid epidemic should include: a) law enforcement b) overdose prevention and c) opioid addiction treatment and prevention.

Law enforcement can often provide the necessary motivation for opioid addicted individuals to change. Similarly, overdose prevention efforts are critically important because lives can be saved with access to overdose rescue medications such as naloxone. I defer to law enforcement and overdose prevention experts to provide their guidance on these important approaches. Since

Alkermes' expertise is in the treatment of opioid addiction, and opioid addiction medications in particular, I will focus the remainder of my written testimony on this topic.

There is an extensive body of research supporting the use of medications and counseling for the treatment of opioid addiction. All opioid addiction treatment medications decrease illicit opioid use and increase retention in treatment.[11]

The three FDA-approved medications for the treatment of opioid addiction all work through the effects they have on opioid receptors in the brain. These are the very same brain cell receptors on which heroin and all prescription opioids have their effect. However, there are significant differences between how the three FDA-approved opioid addiction medications work. Each of these medications has an important role to play in addressing opioid addiction, and each possesses features that make it an indispensible treatment option for individuals addicted to opioids. The three FDA-approved opioid dependence treatment medications are:

- Methadone is a full **opioid agonist**, meaning that it fully stimulates the opioid receptors in a manner similar to heroin and other opioids. As such, it replaces the illicit opioids, freeing the addict from acquiring opioids illegally. Methadone is the first opioid maintenance medication and has been used in the U.S. since the 1960s. Opioid dependent individuals who are treated with methadone are typically required to visit a specially regulated clinic on a near-daily basis and are given methadone under closely supervised conditions. The Drug Enforcement Administration (DEA) Schedule of Controlled Substances lists methadone as a Schedule II controlled substance because it has "a high potential for abuse which may lead to severe psychological or physical dependence."[12] In addition to the supervised administration of methadone, patients are provided with counseling and medical care. There are currently approximately 1,300 opioid treatment programs that administer methadone to about 300,000 patients daily[13].

- Buprenorphine/Naloxone is a **partial opioid agonist**, which means that it partially activates the opioid receptors. As such, buprenorphine/naloxone is also an opioid maintenance treatment. Brand names for buprenorphine/naloxone include SUBOXONE® and ZUBSOLV®; there are also several generic formulations of buprenorphine available. Buprenorphine can be prescribed by any physician once they have fulfilled the federally established educational and credentialing requirements. The DEA Schedule of Controlled Substances lists buprenorphine as a Schedule III controlled substance because it has "a potential for abuse less than substances in Schedules I or II and abuse may lead to moderate or low physical dependence or high psychological dependence."[14] It is estimated that about 1,000,000 people in the U.S. will be treated with buprenorphine this year.[15]

- Long-Acting Injectable Naltrexone (LAI-naltrexone) is an **opioid antagonist**, or blocker.[16] Unlike methadone and buprenorphine, LAI-naltrexone does not activate the opioid receptor at all, but rather works by blocking opioids from activating the opioid receptor.[17] In 2010 LAI-naltrexone was approved by the FDA for the *prevention of relapse to opioid dependence* following detoxification. LAI-naltrexone should be provided as part of a comprehensive treatment program that includes psychosocial support. LAI-naltrexone is non-addictive and non-narcotic and, as such, is not scheduled by the DEA and *is not associated with abuse or diversion for illicit use*. LAI-naltrexone is also FDA-approved for the treatment of alcohol dependence. The brand name for LAI-naltrexone is VIVITROL® (naltrexone for extended-release injectable suspension) and our company, Alkermes, Inc., is the manufacturer of this medication. I provide additional information about LAI-naltrexone later in this testimony.

The two opioid maintenance treatments, methadone and buprenorphine/naloxone, are currently the primary medications used in America today to treat opioid dependence. The number of individuals treated with either methadone or buprenorphine/naloxone increased from approximately 230,000 people in 2003, to more than 1,300,000 individuals in 2014. This five-fold increase is a dramatic development with significant public health implications. For many patients addicted to heroin and other opioids, these opioid maintenance therapies are appropriate treatments and there should be no shame or stigma associated with them. It is also important to recognize that opioid maintenance therapy should not be the only treatment offered to opioid dependent individuals.

The recent growth over the past ten years has introduced some important public health issues. First, there has not been adequate attention paid to how individuals currently maintained on opioid maintenance therapies can be successfully transitioned off of these medications. As early as the 1970s it was shown the termination of opioid maintenance therapy leads to relapse for the vast majority of patients.[18] Consequently, guidelines are urgently needed for identifying which patients need life-long maintenance therapy, and which patients are candidates for transitioning from such treatment. As importantly, guidance is needed concerning best practices for the prevention of relapse for those patients that do end opioid maintenance treatment.

A second significant is the growing problem of illicit diversion of buprenorphine for illicit, non-medical use. According to the DEA, buprenorphine is the third most often seized prescription opioid by law enforcement today and the eighth most often seized illicit drug overall.[19] Methadone, on the other hand, is administered in highly regulated clinics that require close patient supervision. Consequently, while diversion of methadone is a risk, it is a rare event.

In contrast to the opioid maintenance therapies, LAI-naltrexone has no abuse potential or recreational value. Instead of maintaining an addicted individual on an opioid replacement medication, individuals treated with LAI-naltrexone are fully detoxified from all opioids, and then are administered LAI-naltrexone to help prevent relapse to active opioid addiction. With LAI-naltrexone, patients are no longer on any opioids. In addition, since LAI-naltrexone is administered by a health care professional on a monthly basis, the patient is not faced with the challenge of taking medication on a daily basis. Like the other two FDA-approved opioid addiction treatment medications, LAI-naltrexone is not a silver bullet. A patient's motivation, commitment to counseling, and participation in other recovery supports are all important.

In 2012, both the Substance Abuse and Mental Health Services Administration[20] and the White House Office of National Drug Control Policy[21] released publications summarizing key features of LAI-naltrexone including:

- **Not a DEA Scheduled Controlled Substance** – LAI-naltrexone is non-addictive and non-narcotic, and consequently, is not classified in the DEA Schedule of Controlled Substances.

- **Monthly Dosing** – LAI-naltrexone is administered through a gluteal injection once-monthly by a healthcare professional.

- **No Special Credentialing is Required** – Any duly licensed healthcare professional may prescribe and administer LAI-naltrexone; where allowed by state law, physician assistants and nurse practitioners – as well as physicians – may prescribe LAI-naltrexone.

- **No Special Training is Required** – There is no specific training required beyond the directions for use and product information provided in the FDA-approved full prescribing information.

With the approval of LAI-naltrexone for the treatment of opioid dependence, communities have begun to introduce the use of this medication in a variety of settings. For example, in 2008 the Missouri Department of Mental Health became one of the first state agencies to begin using LAI-naltrexone, and since that time, that State has significantly increased its use, especially with alcohol or opioid dependent justice-involved individuals. Additionally, the Missouri Department of Corrections has increased funding for the use of LAI-naltrexone in its prisoner re-entry initiatives and Missouri has also increased the use of LAI-naltrexone in its drug courts. In the past five years, dozens of other states and counties have begun to incorporate LAI-naltrexone as part of their efforts at confronting the opioid problem. Some of these states include Ohio, Texas, Michigan, Pennsylvania, Massachusetts, Illinois, California, Washington, New Jersey, New York, Wisconsin, Florida, and Maine.[22]

A common factor driving the use of LAI-naltrexone by states and counties has been their need to improve outcomes while reducing costs, especially for addicted individuals who are under criminal justice supervision. Adoption of LAI-naltrexone in drug courts has been encouraged by the National Association of Drug Court Professionals, which was quick to recognize the potential benefits of LAI-naltrexone as a non-addictive, non-narcotic medication that has not been associated with diversion or abuse.[23] There are now at least 30 local drug court programs across the country in which LAI-naltrexone has been incorporated, with more courts announcing plans to include it.[24] Notably, the Ohio legislature recently approved a significant project to evaluate the benefit of LAI-naltrexone and other medications with opioid dependent drug court participants.[25]

To effectively address the problem of heroin and opioid dependence in the country today, an approach that recognizes the value of law enforcement, overdose prevention and *all* FDA-approved opioid addiction treatments is needed. People who are addicted to heroin and other opioids deserve the opportunity to become free of all opioids.

More specifically, the Department of Justice should build upon the innovative work being done in the states, and authorize a multi-state program utilizing all opioid addiction medications to support successful reentry of opioid addicted offenders in drug courts and jails (Bureau of Justice

Assistance), federal prisons and reentry centers (Bureau of Prisons), as well as those on supervised parole/release (Administrative Office of the U.S. Courts). The strategy of incarcerating citizens with opioid dependence in our jails and prisons until their time is served and then abandoning them as they re-enter into society has done nothing to reduce the cycle of recidivism or the spread of addiction. We must confront the heroin and opioid addiction epidemic with a comprehensive, coordinated federal and state response using all available evidenced-based approaches.

Many individuals recovering from opioid addiction can tell you the day, and even the hour, when they took their first step into recovery. With the leadership provided by Congress and the states, it is our hope that we will all be able to look back on today, March 17, 2014, as the day when we fully committed to utilizing all tools available to us in the fight to break the cycle of heroin and opioid addiction.

Notes

[1] Robert F. Forman, Ph.D. submitted the testimony on behalf of Alkermes, Inc. Dr. Forman has an extensive background in treatment of opioid and other addictions, with nearly 40 years of experience as a clinician, researcher, teacher and author. In addition to his position at Alkermes, Inc., Dr. Forman serves on the faculty of McLean Hospital and Harvard University School of Medical's Department of Psychology; and previously he served on the faculty of the University of Pennsylvania School of Medicine's Department of Psychiatry; and the Treatment Research Institute. In addition, Dr. Forman has opened over 20 addiction treatment programs; and written over 60 scientific and professional publications. In 2005, Dr. Forman joined Alkermes where he currently is Director of Professional Relations and Policy.

[2] Center for Disease Control (2011). *Vital Signs: Overdoses of Prescription Opioid Pain Relievers — United States, 1999–2008. Morbidity and Mortality Weekly Report*, U.S. Department of Health and Human Services, Volume 60. Jones CM, Mack KA, Paulozzi LJ. *Pharmaceutical overdose deaths*, United States, 2010. JAMA 2013;309:657-659.

[3] Cicero TJ, Ellis MS, Surrat HL. Effect of abuse-deterrent formulation of OxyContin. *The New England Journal of Medicine*, July 12, 2012. Accessed online March 19, 2014 at: https://news.wustl.edu/news/Pages/24025.aspx

[4] NIDA Community Epidemiology Work Group Report, June 2013. Accessed online March 19, 2014: http://www.drugabuse.gov/about-nida/organization/workgroups-interest-groups-consortia/community-epidemiology-work-group-cewg

[5] Gov. Shumlin's 2014 State of the State Address, January 8, 2014. Accessed online March 19, 2014 at: http://governor.vermont.gov/newsroom-state-of-the-state-speech-2013

[6] Ibid.

[7] NIDA Community Epidemiology Work Group Report, June 2013. Accessed online March 19, 2014: http://www.drugabuse.gov/about-nida/organization/workgroups-interest-groups-consortia/community-epidemiology-work-group-cewg

[7] Ibid.

[9] Stephen W. Patrick; Robert E. Schumacher; Brian D. Benneyworth; Elizabeth E. Krans; Jennifer M. McAllister; Matthew M. Davis. **Neonatal Abstinence Syndrome and Associated Health Care Expenditures: United States, 2000-2009**. *JAMA*, 2012 DOI: 10.1001/JAMA.2012.3951

[10] *Ohio Report:* Massatti, R., Falb, M., Yors, A., Potts, L., Beeghly, C. & Starr, S. (2013, November). *Neonatal abstinence syndrome and drug use among pregnant women in Ohio, 2004-2011*. Columbus, OH: Ohio Department of Mental Health and Addiction Services. Accessed on March 19, 2014 online March 19, 2014 at: http://www.healthy.ohio.gov/~/media/HealthyOhio/ASSETS/Files/injury%20prevention/NAS%20Report%20FINAL.ashx . *Tennessee report:* http://health.state.tn.us/MCH/NAS/ *Indiana Report:* http://www.in.gov/attorneygeneral/files/(edit)Winchester_Neonatal_Abstinence_and_Opiate_Prescriptions._12_13_2012_pt.pdf

[11] Substance Abuse and Mental Health Services Administration. (2012). An Introduction to Extended-Release Injectable Naltrexone for the Treatment of People With Opioid Dependence. *Treatment Advisory*, Volume 11, Issue 1. Accessed online March 19, 2014 at: http://store.samhsa.gov/shin/content/SMA12-4682/SMA12-4682.pdf. Thomas et al. Medication-Assisted Treatment With Buprenorphine: Assessing the Evidence. Psychiatric Services in Advance, November 18, 2013; doi: 10.1176/appi.ps.201300256 . Fullerton et al. Medication-Assisted Treatment With Methadone: Assessing the Evidence Psychiatric Services in Advance, November 18, 2013; doi: 10.1176/appi.ps.201300235).

[12] Drug Enforcement Agency Definition of Substance Schedules. Accessed online March 19, 2014 at: http://www.deadiversion.usdoj.gov/schedules/#define

[13] Substance Abuse and Mental Health Services Administration. *Behavioral Health Barometer: United States, 2013*. HHS Publication No. SMA-13-4796. Rockville, MD: Substance Abuse and Mental Health Services Administration, 2013. Accessed online March 19, 2014 at: http://www.samhsa.gov/data/StatesInBrief/2K14/National_BHBarometer.pdf

[14] Drug Enforcement Agency Definition of Substance Schedules. Accessed at: http://www.deadiversion.usdoj.gov/schedules/#define

[15] IMS: SDI's Total Patient Tracker (TPT), Projected Patient Count, Moving Annual Total 2003-2013. Note: The information for buprenorphine and naltrexone are estimates derived from the use of information under license from the following IMS Health information service. IMS expressly reserves all rights, including rights of copying, distribution and republication.

[16] Visit www.VIVITROL.com for important safety and other product information.

[17] The oral formulation of naltrexone is FDA-approved for the treatment of alcohol dependence and the blockade of exogenously administered opioids, but not the treatment of opioid dependence.

[18] Dole, V. and Joseph, H. (1977). Methadone Maintenance - Outcome After Termination. *New York State Journal Of Medicine*. Volume:77 Issue:9, 1409-1412 . Accessed online at March 19, 2014 at: www.ncjrs.gov/App/publications/abstract.aspx?ID=52272 . Also, most recently: Weiss, R. et al. (2011). Adjunctive Counseling During Brief and Extended Buprenorphine-Naloxone Treatment for Prescription Opioid Dependence. *Archives of General Psychiatry*. 68(12):1238-46. Accessed online March 19, 2014 at: http://archpsyc.jamanetwork.com/article.aspx?articleid=1107433
[19] National Forensic Laboratory Information System (NFLIS) 2012 Annual Report. Accessed online March 19, 2014 at: https://www.nflis.deadiversion.usdoj.gov/DesktopModules/ReportDownloads/Reports/NFLIS2012AR.pdf
[20] Substance Abuse and Mental Health Services Administration. (2012). An Introduction to Extended-Release Injectable Naltrexone for the Treatment of People With Opioid Dependence. *Treatment Advisory*, Volume 11, Issue 1. Accessed online March 19, 2014 at: http://store.samhsa.gov/shin/content/SMA12-4682/SMA12-4682.pdf
[21] White House Office of National Drug Control Policy. Healthcare Brief: Medication-Assisted Treatment of Opioid Addiction. September 2012. Accessed online December 21, 2012 at: http://www.whitehouse.gov/sites/default/files/ondcp/recovery/medication_assisted_treatment_9-21-2012L.pdf
[22] For a full-listing of state and county initiatives utilizing VIVITROL in drug courts and other publicly funded settings, see the VIVITROL Public Policy Directory, August 2013 available from Alkermes, Inc.
[23] NADCP. Huddleston, W. *Buprenorphine diversion and its implication for drug courts.* National Association of Drug Court Professionals All Rise magazine, pp. 13-14. Accessed online at: http://www.nadcp.org/sites/default/files/nadcp/Spring%20'12%20All%20Rise%20Magazine%20Final.pdf?q=sites/default/files/nadcp/Spring%20'12%20All%20Rise%20Magazine%20Final.pdf . National Association of Drug Court Professionals. Quality Improvement for Drug Courts: Evidence Based Standards. (2008). Accessed at: http://www.ndci.org/publications/monograph-series/quality-improvement-drug-courts . NADCP. FDA Approves First Once-Monthly, Non-Narcotic, Non-Addictive Medicine for Opioid Dependence. Accessed online at: http://nadcp.org/node/605 . NADCP. Adult Drug Court Best Practice Standards, volume 1. (2013). Accessed online at: http://www.nadcp.org/sites/default/files/nadcp/AdultDrugCourtBestPracticeStandards.pdf For example, see page 44. NADCP. Honorable Judge Alan Blankenship and Pam Sams. Hopeless No More. All Rise, Spring 2013. pp. 20-21 accessed online at: http://nadcp.org/sites/default/files/nadcp/magazine/spring2013/index.html
[24] Davis, K. *Vivitrol is the new hope for solving opiate addiction. San Diego City Beat.* January 30, 2013. Accessed online at: http://www.sdcitybeat.com/sandiego/article-11438-vivitrol-is-the-new-hope-for-solving-opiate-addiction.html Also, see VIVITROL Public Policy Directory, August 2013 available from Alkermes.
[25] See FOX19 Investigates: A magic shot for addiction? October 30, 2013 Accessed online at: http://www.fox19.com/story/23827503/a-magic-shot-for-addiction-vivitrol-and-our-heroin-epidemic

http://projectlazarus.org/about-lazarus/project-lazarus-model

The Project Lazarus Model (an edited synopsis)

.....reversing Wilkes County's epidemic of drug overdoses.

http://projectlazarus.org/about-lazarus/project-lazarus-model

The Project Lazarus public health model is based on the premises that drug overdose deaths are preventable and that all communities are ultimately responsible for their own health.

The model components:

(1) community activation and coalition building.....in responding to overdoses among law enforcement, physicians, and pain patients.

(2) monitoring and epidemiologic surveillance

(3) prevention of overdoses through medical education and other means

(4) use of rescue medication to reverse overdoses by community members

Naloxone OD Antidote: used in programs all over the world to effectively reverse opioid overdoses.

Naloxone: The Second Chance: important tool for empowering communities to protect their health.

Naloxone: There are two kinds of naloxone, one that you can squirt up someone's nose and another that can be injected through clothing into a muscle.

(5) evaluation of project components. The last four steps operate in a cyclical manner, with community advisory boards playing the central role in developing and designing each aspect of the intervention.

Attention: The Centers for Disease Control and Prevention (CDC) reports more than 10,000 reversals of overdoses with naloxone by non-medical bystanders!

The Wilkes County Experience ....reversing Wilkes County's epidemic of drug overdoses.

The CPI approach is modeled on a highly successful Wilkes County overdose prevention program known as Project Lazarus. The program began with a series of public meetings organized by the Wilkes County Health Department to heighten community awareness of the county's exceptionally high rate of mortalities attributable to overdoses of prescribed opioid pain relievers. In 2008, Project Lazarus, a secular, non-profit drug overdose prevention program, was formed to develop and disseminate a set of strategic action plans for the community and tool kits and medical training for local medical care providers to address opioid misuse and abuse.

Wilkes County generated a 47% reduction in the overdose death rate from 2009 to 2010. More recent data show that the overdose death rate in Wilkes County decreased by 69% between 2009 and 2011, from 46.0 to 14.4 per 100,000 per year (see graph below), even as the level of opioid prescribing remained above the state average. Substance abuse-related ED admissions dropped by 15.3% from 2008 to 2010………

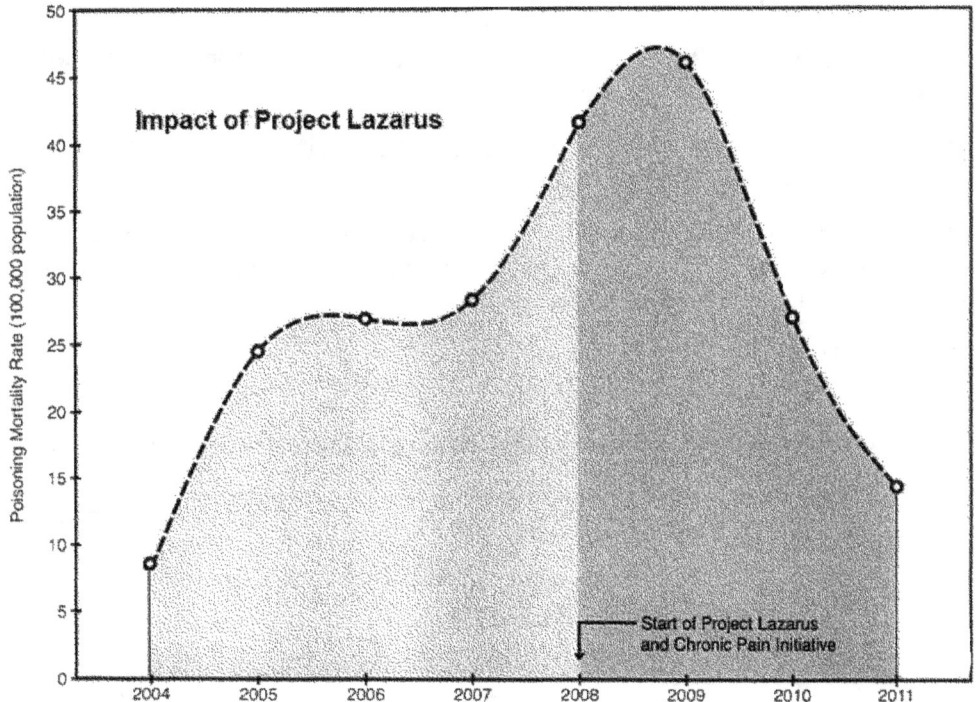

Data from Wilkes County suggest that the results of Project Lazarus became apparent within two years of its initiation, and that strong effects were apparent by the third year. The Project Lazarus is a model of enhanced and coordinated empowerment in responding to overdoses among law enforcement, physicians, and pain patients.

http://projectlazarus.org/about-lazarus/project-lazarus-model

THE REMEDY...........Naloxone, the OD Antidote

Naloxone: The Second Chance Drug

***Naloxone (also called Narcan) is the antidote that reverses an opioid overdose. It has been used in abulances and hospitals for decades to reverse overdose.

***It's legal and has been approved by the Food and Drug Administration (FDA). It works by neutralizing the opioids in your system and helping you breathe again.

***Naloxone only works if a person has opioids in their system; the medication doesn't work on other drugs. You can't get high from it and it is safe for nearly everyone. It has been used in programs all over the world to effectively reverse opioid overdoses.

***There are two kinds of naloxone, one that you can squirt up someone's nose and another that can be injected through clothing into a muscle.

***Project Lazarus provides naloxone for FREE through Brame Huie Pharmacy in North Wilkesboro.

***The Centers for Disease Control and Prevention (CDC) reports more than 10,000 reversals of overdoses with naloxone by non-medical bystanders!

***Naloxone is also an important tool for empowering communities to protect their health. Reviving an overdose victim can be a very powerful motivator to help people change their behaviors.

GET ONLINE TO FIND: fact sheet on naloxone shows examples of how naloxone is empowering.

Check out these great resources from the Harm Reduction Coalition, including educational materials, manuals, best practice documents, case studies, research and more.

Attention Prescribers and Committee Members !!

The strategy created by Project Lazarus includes the following understanding and actions:

*community-level response to prescription opioid use problems must address pain and abuse/addiction simultaneously.

*centers around community activation and a strong coalition of partners who have an active interest in preventing prescription overdose deaths.

* capitalizes on using existing data sources to provide perspectives on fatal and nonfatal overdoses and serves as a mechanism to evaluate interventions.

http://projectlazarus.org/about-lazarus/project-lazarus-model

* multiple levels of prevention efforts and community-based education are intended to reach medical care providers as well as pain patients and nonmedical drug users without exacerbating stigma.

* School-based prevention education targets vulnerable populations and aims to shift general patterns of substance abuse. The provision of take-home naloxone acknowledges that prevention efforts can fail or take years to have effect and that overdose deaths can be prevented in the community.

*Target communities for replicating the Project Lazarus model include those with high prescription opioid unintentional poisoning rates and some degree of community awareness and coalition building capacity.

*Target communities for replicating the Project Lazarus model may include those with high prescription overdose rates, some degree of community awareness and coalition building capacity.

*The presence of a motivated community organizer, support from the medical establishment, and strong data utilization practices are key components for replication.

*The Project Lazarus model has been evaluated in peer-reviewed publications. See the evidence online.
* See presentation by Bill Matthews, PA on Community-based opioid overdose prevention.

http://projectlazarus.org/about-lazarus/project-lazarus-model

http://projectlazarus.org/about-lazarus/project-lazarus-model

The Project Lazarus Model

The Project Lazarus public health model is based on the premises that drug overdose deaths are preventable and that all communities are ultimately responsible for their own health. The model components: (1) community activation and coalition building, (2) monitoring and epidemiologic surveillance, (3) prevention of overdoses through medical education and other means, (4) use of rescue medication to reverse overdoses by community members, and (5) evaluation of project components. The last four steps operate in a cyclical manner, with community advisory boards playing the central role in developing and designing each aspect of the intervention.

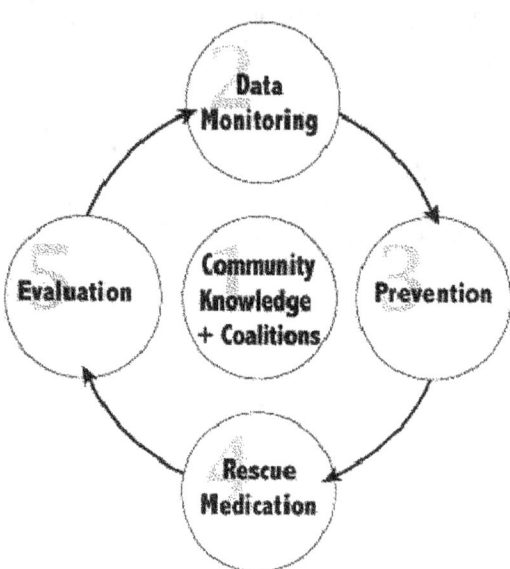

Read more details of the Project Lazarus Model in scientific papers or our recent results.

20 March 2014
To whom it may concern,

My name is Heather Bryant, I am a 42 yr old woman living in Northern Vermont. I am writing to share my experience of using narcotics at a young age, what happened, how I got away from them, and what I feel successful treatment entails.

I grew up in a small town in Northern California called, Crescent City. This town was a logging and fishing community when I was growing up there in the 1980's. It is now what is known as a Prison Town. Pelican Bay State Prison, the highest maximum security prison in the entire state of CA was built 3 miles out of town. It was a promise to boost the economy! The opposite happened. The industries dried up, the downtown died, the drug use has escalated as the population increased with the addition of families of the inmates. Being a Correctional Officer is the most sought after form of employment.

Crescent City already had a reputation of high crystal meth use, also known as the poor mans' cocaine. The drug is called this because, it cost 1/3 the price of cocaine and lasts 3x as long, anywhere from 6-12 hrs. It was introduced to me at the age of 15. I became addicted to it over time. Mainly from hanging out with people who used it. It didn't seem that bad.
I could still go to school, and work, and it kept me trim. Alas, it took its toll on my body, and my life. I stopped using when I moved to Santa Rosa, CA and lived with people who did not use it, and thought it was gross. Unfortunately some of my friends and family members were not so lucky. They never stopped using, and after 20yrs, are phantoms of the people I once knew and loved. During this time, the 1980's, meth was primarily a West Coast Drug.

Eventually, my travels took me to NYC, and later VT. I arrived in VT in 1998. In the 15 years I have lived here, I have watched the drug make its way across the country and further. People say Hawaii is overridden with it and the crime rate has escalated.

In my opinion and experience, the best treatment for drug abuse is first, to get away from it. This often requires the participation and support of loved ones. It is VITAL to be around people who do not use drugs, and enjoy doing other things. Once you can get clear, and back in touch with yourself, you are able to remember what brings you Joy!!! Real Joy!!!

I don't feel replacing one drug with another, legal, prescribed, etc, is an effective answer to getting Vermont's addicts off drugs. That's just another way to get addicted to something else...and once addicted to some other drug it's easy to get back into the same routine. The REAL answer is FUN!! This is why most kids start using in the FIRST place.
To have FUN and FEEL GOOD!!

In my experience, I believe if we can encourage recreation in healthy forms and truthful, straight up drug education, we may be able to head off the addiction in young people. We can help the addict in a similar manner. Don't just prescribe addicts more drugs. It may look good for a while, but more drugs are just more of the same stuff just in a different form. This doesn't help.

I have been introduced to recreational therapists. These are people who do NOT prescribe more drugs to handle addiction or depression, but who work one on one with individuals, helping them to identify what brings them joy in their lives and in the process of doing this interest or activity with the addict, help establish what may have been forgotten or never learned in the first place,

Please, strive to put funding in this non-drug area of treatment along with honest drug education and end the revolving door of drug use, abuse, and addiction.

Thank you for your time, consideration and participation.

Sincerely,
Heather Bryant

Dear Sen. Leahy,

Back in 1982 I witnessed a near fatal heroin overdose by a man who became my first brother in-law. He later died of AIDS and we have since made HIV a livable disease. All these years later, we have made progress on gay rights which back then was another taboo subject and initially thought of as the only demographic who could get AIDS. Yet we are still bewildered about our drug problem in America. In fact, it seems to have become more mainstream. Some people are against having methadone clinics in their town; although perhaps next to a school isn't an ideal location.

We have also made little progress on minimum wages and cost of living. If more people earned more and had a better outlook on life, perhaps drug use would decrease. We lack support for people recently out of jail or in other bad situations: recently widowed or laid off during a bad economy for example. How can government help its citizens? Our response so far has been mainly to put people in jail after crimes are committed and not get involved in family matters. If social workers were involved in domestic disputes as much as the police, maybe we would have a less volatile society.

We need to be more caring of our citizens and less afraid of their drugs. We should put all options on the table and see what doesn't work. The worst that can happen is the reality we now have.

Steve Handley
Waitsfield

To Senator Leahy and concerned members

I have worked as an LADC in Vermont since 2002 in schools and in an agency as well as private practice. I've talked to school administration, doctors, Court Diversion and Probation about this growing problem but felt I was not heard. I gave up trying to be heard. I don't feel Drug Evaluations are valid without valid urine screens. There are not enough labs that can do that with any degree of accuracy. Burlington Labs is one of the few and are not expensive but they could not find an office to host them to do urine screen collections in Addison County. They tried to do it at the Turning Point in Middlebury but the stigma was too much for the AA members so they were told to leave. A clinic or public building for this would really help. This would make a difference not only in the accountability for drug testing but also for alcohol use since this lab runs tests for ETG (ethylgluconoride) which is the enzyme for digesting alcohol detected in the body several days after consumption. This small effort could make a big difference for our youth and anyone on probation or Court Diversion who has any kind of drug/alcohol related offense. The pot smoking culture in this state has not been willing to see how the very strong level of THC in pot these days quickly leads to developing a high tolerance and can (not always) lead to other drug use. Mostly however, I believe the rising opiate abuse is from irresponsible prescriptions from doctors and dentists who will hand out entire bottles of pills instead of saying take two aspirin and call me in the morning. They do not want the call the next month when the client is addicted. They do not want to follow up on these issues.

One last comment, but I think very promising, is the introduction of a new technique that I believe could prove extremely effective in the treatment of opiate addiction in a very short time. Please check it out on YouTube "Faster EFT heroin addiction", if you have any interest at all in a short term inexpensive proven treatment that is easy to learn and get trained in. EFT has been validated as a best practice. This advanced form of tapping is called FasterEFT and has been used in the rehabilitation centers called Habilitat in Hawaii and Oklahoma for heroin addiction. It consists of tapping on the meridian system while bringing up cravings and related feelings associated with the addiction. I am being trained in it at this time but so far have found it useful in cigarette addiction, sex addictions and food addictions. It is truly remarkable, quick and easy. I think it could have an impressive impact in Methadone clinics or treatment centers in Vermont as well as in agencies all over. It addresses the cravings as well as the underlying issues. Thank you for taking a look at it.

One last comment in regards to the addiction field. Opiate addicted clients need support more than a one hour per week due to their high need for case management. It is not realistic to expect therapists in private practice to be successful with this. These clients usually need wrap around services.

Thank you for listening

Julianne Holland MA., LADC

My name is Lynne Klamm; I have lived in Rutland my entire life, raised my children here and am now lucky enough to watch my grandchild live and grow here. I also work for the State as a Field Director for the Agency of Human Services. I have worked for the State for almost 34 years in various capacities, including for the Department of Corrections and Family Services. I am part of Project Vision and was able to attend the hearing that was held in Rutland this week.

Rutland is a great place to live and work. My oldest son has left the area a couple different times and lived in Colorado, Massachusetts and Florida. He always comes back because he says there is no other place like it. Sometimes the depth of the opiate problem makes it easy to forget that most of the people who live and work here are not addicts, but are hard-working folks who understand what Rutland and Vermont have to offer and who choose to stay here.

At a Federal level, when looking at the opiate problem, I think one has to acknowledge that there is some level of accountability with the medical profession. They are the ones who prescribe narcotic drugs. This is often how an addictions begins. When I was a probation officer a few years back, I had a bright, personable young man on my caseload, who had lost a good job and family support because of his drug use. When I asked him how it started he told me he had hurt his back while playing softball and had gone to the Dr. and gotten Percocet. Really? What happened to ice packs and hot showers? We cannot support a culture that says the drugs are the answer when you are uncomfortable. Prescribers have to take responsibility for this. Maybe they are the ones who have to just start saying "no" to drugs. We do not need Zohydro. In my opinion, that is just big pharmaceutical money talking.

A couple of weeks ago, on Town Meeting Day, I went to our local mall. When I came out, at 2 PM, I observed a drug deal taking place right next to my car. The "buyer" was a young man who had gone to school with my daughter. The "sellers" were a young white female and a young black man. This is an all too common sight and one that occurs out in the open fairly regularly if you know what to look for. There is no fear on the part of these folks, only on the part of those of us who watch it happening around us. While watching scenes like this angers me, I also feel sad for those people who are caught in its grip and who see no other options in their lives. Buying or selling or both never have good outcomes. How awful that life must be.

There are several things that I think can be done to assist in this fight:
1) Recall Zohydro before it hits the streets;
2) Adjust managed care/Medicaid regulations to allow for longer than 15 day stays in residential treatment; that is barely enough time for someone to detox and certainly nowhere near enough time to address the underlying addictive thinking;
3) Mandate physician participation in annual drug training as well as use of the electronic pharmacy records;
4) Create programs within schools to support students whose parents are addicts; we know that home-visiting and outreach are effective community strategies so let's use them;
5) Increase funding for low –cost, big-bang-for-your-buck programs, like Recovery Centers; their budgets are small but their impact is not; provide enough money so that they can have full-time staff.

None of these ideas cost a lot of money but all would be a part of the plan to address this public health issue. Thank you, Senator Leahy so much for your support and for your unwavering representation of the citizens of Vermont.

Lynne Klamm
Agency of Human Services
Field Director
Rutland County
802-786-5952
Fax: 802-789-0088
Addison County
802-388-5385
Fax: 802-388-4665

Dear Senator,

I would like to add my voice to the concerned people of Vermont at what is being done to counter drug abuse in our state. Although many solutions have been tried over the decades, there is one program that attains real results everywhere it is in action. This is the Drug Free World Campaign :

http://www.drugfreeworld.org/home.html

I urge to please see what has been done successfully around the world to fight the scourge of drugs with this campaign.

Yours,

A concerned Vermonter and Father of 2.

Julian Partridge

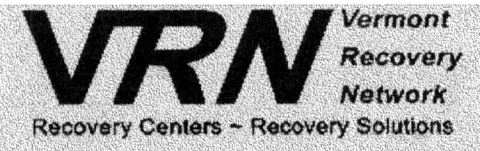

Vermont Recovery Network
200 Olcott Drive
White River Junction, VT 05001
vtrecoverynetwork@gmail.com
www.vtrecoverynetwork.org
802-738-8998

Vermont's Recovery System — preventing multigenerational cycles of Addiction

Governor Shumlin was right to encourage state officials to respond to drug and alcohol addiction as a chronic disease, which we should address with treatment and recovery support, rather than only punishment and incarceration. Vermont is in the enviable position of being the only state in the country with a statewide, peer-based recovery system that is capable of responding with supports appropriate to the chronic nature of addictive disease.

The Governor's budget this year includes a request for additional state resources to develop a more robust recovery system. Moving people out of expensive justice services into recovery supports will also benefit from the development of Federal funding streams that support this paradigm shift. Vermont's forming recovery support system is beginning to document its ability to prevent multi-generational cycles of addiction, providing a solution to recidivism for those in corrections and treatment.

Of the chronic diseases we respond to, addictive disease costs our state the most. Our costs related to the healthcare system, justice system, corrections, and social services systems make this the most expensive problem we face—and this doesn't count the human costs. http://www.casacolumbia.org/newsroom/op-eds/how-permanently-reduce-state-medicaid-and-prison-costs Individual lives are lost to cycles of addiction. Addiction undermines families and causes incredible suffering for all involved.

Vermont has become a national leader in utilizing researched community prevention approaches, but until we can develop the infrastructure for breaking the inter-generational cycles of addiction that plague so many families, these efforts will continue to be undermined. Opiate addiction has become rampant. Youngsters growing up with role models who use substances as a solution to life problems have experienced earlier and earlier patterns of first use, a situation that has been documented to increase the likelihood of addictions. People in the grip of addictions continue to make the bad choices that keep them stuck in the revolving doors at courts and corrections departments. Vermont Department of Corrections has estimated that 85% of their populations are incarcerated as a direct result of alcohol and drug use; many of them repeat offenders. **Until we address the underlying cause—people with addictions who have not yet taken responsibility for rebuilding their lives—the societal costs of addictions will continue to escalate.**

Vermont has begun the practice of using the crisis of an arrest as a motivator for encouraging people with lower level crimes to seek treatment and recovery supports as a way to avoid becoming entangled in the justice system. Those people with addictions who are successful in these efforts require ongoing recovery supports to help prevent the cycles of recidivism. It would be simplistic to suggest that providing only treatment will bend this curve. We need to expand the webs of community support for those leaving justice system interventions and custody. We are beginning to be able to engage them in communities of recovery instead of the communities of addiction that fuel the cycles of recidivism.

Many of the participants in Burlington, Vermont's initial experiments with rapid interventions were referred to the Turning Point Center of Chittenden County for recovery coaching after being identified as having trouble with drugs and alcohol, and therefore potential candidates for direct immersion in recovery. Burlington State's Attorney T.J. Donovan's glowing report on the effectiveness of what was first called "rapid arraignment" included many of the same people who provided the basis for an independent study we contracted for on the effectiveness of recovery coaching.

Vermont Recovery Network (VRN) and our evaluators at Evidence Based Solutions (EBS) have developed a tool for documenting the effectiveness of recovery coaching. It tracks the participants' use of treatment, justice, medical, and social services over time and documents progress in developing self sufficiency through the use of a Self Sufficiency Matrix (SSM). The SSM was developed by the Pennsylvania State Department of Health, Bureau of Drug and Alcohol Services Case Management Workgroup (Pennsylvania Department of Health, 1999). It assesses an individual's level of supports across a number of domains including housing, childcare, education, vocational, employment, basic needs, transportation, substance abuse treatment, legal, mental health, physical health, family/social, and life skills. Results are used to develop an evolving recovery plan, addressing highest areas of need first.

The SSM has demonstrated that over time, individuals who take part in recovery coaching experience **statistically significant increases in their recovery capital** and develop increased social connections. Connections with new peer groups are critical to achieving ongoing recovery. The findings have also documented positive changes in the lives of these people in recovery. Their **statistically significant reduced use of treatment, justice, medical, and social services over time** indicate the potential for significant savings and demonstrate the need for broader study and increasing the use of this approach. https://vtrecoverynetwork.org/PDF/VRN_RC_eval_report.pdf

Recovery coaching is a promising practice; all eleven VRN centers have coaching teams. **We view recovery coaching as a more formal and intensive version of the peer-to-peer supports that our centers have always provided.** The formal relationship between a person in recovery and a coach has provided us with an opportunity to document the outcomes that result from supporting someone in taking responsibility for changing their life and finding a personal pathway to recovery.

Relevant facts: Over the last 8 years, 1/3 of the people who utilize recovery centers (N=8,023 surveys) have moved directly from substance use to recovery without the need for treatment, but recovery services receive only 1% of the current addictions budget. [Note: The nature of our services doesn't match current fee-for-service Medicaid reimbursement approaches.]

Last year, recovery centers hosted 13,524 guests who made 168,369 visits across the network's eleven recovery centers. Centers collected 1,152 "Participant Surveys" from a representative sample of guests. Visitors come, on average, 12.45 times per month. We serve more men (55%) than women (45%). Our average visitor is just over 40. Centers have many occasional visitors; an *average* of more than 100 regulars who come for 2 or 3 visits a week, and a small revolving population of high-utilization visitors coming daily until their lives stabilize. Our visitors get their lives in order, find jobs, find housing, repair the damage caused by addictive behaviors, and function in recovery as productive members of their communities – often for the first time in their lives.

Upon initiating their use of recovery centers' supports, 26% of individuals report being on probation or parole and 24% report being released from probation or parole. Interestingly, while 54% report criminal incidents/ involvement before involvement at recovery centers, **only 8% report new criminal incidents/involvement after becoming involved with recovery centers**.

Seventy-five percent of our guests report current or past participation in mental health services and/or supports. With respect to treatment utilization, approximately 72% of survey respondents reported receiving substance abuse treatment in the past; 29% had been in treatment during the previous 30 days; and 27% reported never having attended treatment. Documented increases in collaboration with treatment providers during the last year tracks with this increase in treatment utilization, but we also continue to demonstrate the power of peer recovery for supporting people not interested or able to participate in treatment.

Vermont's Recovery System — A Solution to Recidivism

The federal government is supporting the development of recovery-oriented systems of care (ROSC) across the country because of growing evidence that implementing peer recovery support services saves money and helps more people achieve and maintain recovery. Treatment is a short-term event that is helpful to many people. However, successfully maintaining a lifelong recovery lifestyle often requires ongoing, community-based recovery supports.

Vermont is recognized as a national leader in the recovery movement because our network of eleven recovery centers has evolved into a *recovery system* that is outstanding for employing evidence-based programs and promising practices; capturing definitive outcome data; and – importantly – providing systematic peer oversight. For example, network outcome data studies on recovery coaching have documented reductions in the utilization of costly services such as emergency rooms, hospitals, courts, and corrections, while increasing use of primary care physicians.

The Vermont Recovery Network, in collaboration with the Vermont Department of Health, provides oversight for the centers, which developed and agreed to abide by Standards for the Provision of Recovery Services. Our Network peer review committee audits each center, examining policies & procedures, adherence to ethical guidelines, organizational health, and compliance with outcome data standards. Network committees have developed a broad menu of recovery services and performance evaluation measures. The Network has formed a relationship with the Connecticut Certification Board to participate in developing standards for certifying recovery coaches. The Network has also been providing ongoing training for coaches to enhance their capabilities as new needs and concerns emerge among Vermont's addicted populations.

Rising to the Challenge Vermont's Opiate Problem

Vermont recovery centers have been seeing increasing numbers of visitors looking for physicians who can prescribe Buprenorphine or methadone. These visitors report that they are in recovery, but are buying Buprenorphine on the street until they can find a willing physician. We take the position that our visitors are in recovery when they say they are. This era is bringing new people into our recovery centers who are looking to avoid the discomfort of withdrawal symptoms but have not yet realized how rich recovery can be. In many cases, they have not yet made a personal commitment to medication compliance and giving up the use of alcohol and other drugs.

We are committed to making recovery available to all who seek support in changing their lives, BUT we need to maintain safe, supportive environments for people on ALL paths to recovery. *The influx of opiate users beginning their recovery journey has made it imperative that we have more trained recovery workers on site every hour a center is open to keep our centers safe.* We identified the need to develop trained staff to help these visitors and applied for SAMHSA's Targeted Capacity Expansion Peer to Peer funding to help address this high need population with opiate problems.

Pathways to Recovery

As a result of our demonstrated success in providing recovery supports, the Vermont Recovery Network received Federal funding to implement a pilot project, Pathways to Recovery, which will provide support for Vermonters in opiate treatment. People in opiate treatment have not had consistent access to welcoming peer recovery groups and recovery support services. All of Vermont's recovery centers now host ½ time "Pathway Guides," paid by VRN, who are working with opiate treatment providers and receiving referrals for one-on-one support and/or facilitated peer recovery support. Pathway Guides will increase available staff time at each participating recovery center and demonstrate the benefit of providing expanded peer recovery support for people in recovery from opiate addictions. Because this grant doesn't cover supervision or office space, Vermont recovery centers are stretching already tight budgets to support this program. These part-time experts on the recovery process will help people seeking support for opiate addiction, but because their employment is limited to accomplishing VRN's grant objectives, they will be unable to meet the recovery centers' general staffing needs.

Our experience with providing recovery support has demonstrated that recovery centers help visitors reduce recidivism and become productive members of their communities. Our approach to providing information and peer support for people recovering from addictive disease helps them take responsibility for managing their lives with this chronic health condition, just as people with diabetes, asthma, or heart problems have traditionally benefitted from information and targeted recovery support. Our Pathway Guides will function as ambassadors of recovery and help people in medication-assisted treatment to develop their own vision of how their lives could become more comfortable and satisfying in ongoing recovery. We help people regain their enthusiasm for life.

We have already developed introductions to various recovery approaches such as: All Recovery meetings, Making Recovery Easier groups, and our pilot Recovery is the Solution groups, which answer the question, "Why would I want recovery?" Recovery centers host these groups to introduce participants to others in recovery, helping them to create their own webs of recovery support.

The Pathways to Recovery project will make it possible for our team to refine these recovery approaches, while working with those providing medication-assisted treatment. Guides will coordinate with treatment professionals to determine mutually agreeable ways to introduce people in treatment to personally directed recovery approaches. Many providers and centers have regularly scheduled visits where center representatives introduce themselves and the recovery supports available in recovery centers to treatment clients. Increased staff support will allow us to expand these efforts.

Enhancing our Network's capacity to Realize Our Vision

Vermont's established peer-led, statewide recovery services delivery system has made substantial progress but has been stymied by the following impediments:

1) Insufficient resources for providing the recovery supports we have developed;
2) Insufficient resources for refining and implementing recovery practice guidelines and Recovery Services Standards we have already developed;
3) Insufficient resources for managing and distributing funds from VRN for the benefit of the individual recovery centers.

In order to address this challenge we have again sought funding from SAMHSA to expand VRN's infrastructure to operate more effectively and efficiently, better meet workforce development needs for peer recovery support services, and to promote the integration of peer services into primary care and behavioral health settings. The results we have already achieved with the administrator for our Pathways to Recovery Opiate program have demonstrated the potential for growth that can be expected from having an expanded capacity to manage funding for recovery services from a central point of contact. We believe that this additional funding will lead to significant progress in expanding the Vermont Recovery Network's administrative and fiscal infrastructure. This statewide enhancement project will enable our Vermont recovery system to: negotiate for increased funding opportunities with other entities, disburse funds, expand capacity to collect outcome data, report outcomes, further develop protocols, assure uniformity in recovery services delivery, refine peer governance and oversight structure, and refine the collaborative peer review process of our Provider Standards for Recovery Services.

With or without this funding, Vermont's recovery system is poised to provide significant changes in the long-term outcomes of people seeking recovery. Our system has demonstrated its capacity for delivering low-cost, cost-saving services, but the unique nature of peer services requires the development of reimbursement mechanisms that are consistent with the provision of recovery supports in anonymous and welcoming environments. Conceivably, this will happen through health-care reform approaches that manage costs for large populations utilizing capitated rates, but we would be remiss if we didn't request support in looking out for potential opportunities that support the realization of this vision. Although we have not yet been able to fully refine our approaches, or document completely the results that can be achieved by our peer recovery supports delivery system, we stand ready to advance from the efficacy we have shown and the promise we have demonstrated.

Challenges to Realizing Our Vision

Vermont's recovery centers were originally conceived as "drop-in centers," or safe places people could visit to connect with others in recovery and begin the process of redefining themselves as people who do not use drugs and alcohol. However, in recent years, the centers have evolved into multifaceted operations providing an increasingly sophisticated array of peer-support programs and educational opportunities. The centers are a front door to Vermont's treatment system, as well as a destination after treatment. In some cases, centers offer support until treatment is available; in others, recovery supports offer a direct path to a life in recovery.

Unfortunately, our funding has not kept pace with the growth of our programs. Funding that was adequate for a drop-in center employing a part-time director, maybe a part-time volunteer coordinator, and a crew of volunteers is not nearly sufficient for today's far more professional and sophisticated recovery centers. Currently, center directors must simultaneously work with high-need individuals; manage and schedule volunteers; run recovery support groups; maintain facilities; raise funds; and coordinate, train, and maintain recovery coaching programs—all while maintaining collaborative relationships with community partners. The turnover is higher among center directors than it should be because of low pay, burnout, and frustration with limitations on their ability to function. We are losing volunteers because we lack sufficient staff to schedule, train, and honor this volunteer workforce that is critical to our success.

In spite of these serious constraints, our centers have succeeded in expanding their reach and establishing innovative peer support programs for guests seeking recovery solutions. When limited, temporary funding has been available; our centers have launched pilot programs, such as recovery coaching, to demonstrate the effectiveness of recovery support services. Although these programs have stretched the centers' capacity, the results have been promising, and collaborators in the community who make referrals to these programs respond enthusiastically to them.

But without proper levels of staffing – especially supervisory and coordinator support – centers face difficulties in sustaining the broad range of recovery supports we have already demonstrated are effective. We have repeatedly demonstrated that people once viewed as hopeless can succeed when exposed to peer recovery services, but we lack staffs of recovery workers to provide the services we have developed. Trained recovery support workers move on to other opportunities when supervisory support is lacking and training funds are not available. Employees are donating many hours of service to keep our system afloat.

Millions of dollars are spent each year to make sure that people who suffer from the effects of addictive disease get treatment and sufficient medications. Likewise, millions of dollars are spent on our medical system, justice system, and other human services programs whose caseloads are filled with people stuck in addictive lifestyles. But we have not devoted resources to recovery supports that would assure that these people move on and *maintain* productive lives in recovery. In short, because we have not made a proper investment in recovery supports, we have been losing a significant part of the much larger investments we were already making.

Realizing Our Vision

We envision recovery centers having full-time directors, volunteer coordinators, and recovery coach coordinators. In our vision, permanent staffs would recruit and sustain volunteer workers and coaches, creating stronger, more highly skilled volunteer teams and coaching programs. A more robust recovery workforce would provide a broader array of recovery supports, a stronger community intervention capacity, and stronger partnerships with treatment and prevention providers.

We envision fully supported and recognized volunteers who would stay with us longer, perhaps moving on to coaching or facilitating support groups. Mentored coaching teams would support coaches who stay longer and become more skilled in what they do. Formal interventions orchestrated by recovery workers would help more people understand their need for recovery, and possibly treatment. Staff and volunteers would provide ongoing outreach to community partners, as well as to individuals and families needing recovery supports. These more robust teams would create partnerships with community prevention efforts, perform more interventions, and support youth and families with a true Resiliency and Recovery-Oriented System of Care.

Most important of all, our guests would have access to a rich variety of recovery supports offered by teams of skilled recovery support workers. Broader menus of recovery supports would reach more people who would then successfully maintain their recoveries. These recovering people would establish ongoing peer supports, find stable housing, heal their family relationships, become better parents, secure jobs or more schooling, improve their health, resolve their legal matters—all to become healthy, contributing members of their communities.

We stand at the Turning Point with opportunities for significant improvements in combatting the impacts that addictions have across our human services systems. We hope you share our vision, and will help us achieve it.

Thank you for the opportunity to express my thoughts on the opioid and heroin problem in Vermont and Rutland in particular. I attended the Senate Judiciary hearing in Rutland on March 20 and was impressed with the intent of solutions based testimony. Those in attendance were very impressed with Mary Alice McKenzie's presentation about the effect of hard drugs and children.

I would like to echo Mary Alice's perspective. I am the Executive Director of the Boys & Girls Club of Rutland County and we see the effect of heroin and opiates on our young members on a daily basis. Last month, our club in Brandon had a major heroin bust 5 houses away from the Brandon Boys & Girls Club. The mother of one of members, a seven year old boy, was charged felony possession of cocaine and heroin trafficking. The police found 380 bags of heroin and 32 bags of crack cocaine. The seven year old is now living in New York with his "father" who has a history of drug usage and criminal activity.

The seven year old had been attending the Brandon Boys & Girls Club for 2 years when this happened. The staff never saw him eat a bite of the nightly dinner we serve. I made a point to "share" a meal with him when I was in Brandon and he would then eat 3-5 bites before he lost interest. Whenever a staff person asked him to lower his voice or put stuff away, he would hide under a table for hours-thinking that he had been reprimanded. He would cry when it was time to leave the club and often said that he did not want to go home.

I share his story because we unfortunately see this far too often at our Boys & Girls Club across the state of Vermont. When we gather as an alliance, we share our sad stories of the effects of drugs on our youth, mostly it is behavior- acting out in anger, bullying and isolating. Sometimes it is stealing, sometimes it is suicide. (Brattleboro 2 months ago, and Brandon 8 months ago.)

The parents of our youth that are dealing with addiction cannot parent in a proactive way. Because of their addictions, they are reactive parents and the only time their children get attention is when they get in trouble. This reactive parenting is often in a negative verbal and/or physical form, which in turn lowers the youth's self-esteem and leads them to seek attention in any way they can....and the sad cycle continues from generation to generation.

Mary Alice is correct in saying that community collaboration is the key to breaking this cycle, we need to work together for the sake of the youth who are born with 2 strikes against them (and they are not going to get the benefit of any close calls on that third strike).

In Rutland, Chief Baker is to be commended for initiating "The Vision" project. My hope is that this project will continue for years to come and we will see results one home at a time, one youth at a time.

Thank you.

Larry Bayle
Executive Director
Boys & Girls Club of Rutland County

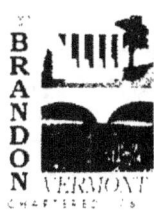

Brandon Police Department
301 Forest Dale Road, Brandon, VT 05733
Tel. (802) 247-0222 Fax (802) 247-0221
Christopher J. Brickell   *Chief of Police*

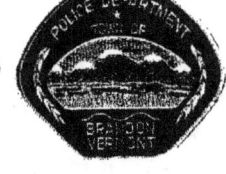

Senator Leahy and members of the Senate Judiciary Committee, I am pleased to be offered the opportunity to address the committee and express my gratitude for your efforts to assist rural communities in Vermont with the struggles of opiate addiction.

At your recent hearing in Rutland Vermont, you heard of the heartbreaking stories of our citizens and families who have suffered with the problem of opiate abuse. It is a reality that we have faced now for several years due to the abundance of illegal drugs available from outside Vermont, and the profit to be made by those who negatively impact our way of life, our family structure, and the lives of Vermonters. We are a small state of hard working resourceful people who have suddenly found ourselves with limited answers as to how to help free our family members from this epic problem. As a result of this problem, accentuated by recent deaths of our citizens, the law enforcement community has looked at ways to collaborate with community partners, educators, substance abuse counselors, health care workers, and anyone else that can join together with us to fight this epidemic. As stated at your hearing this is a problem that requires the efforts of a variety of services and cannot be cured by law enforcement alone.

In my own community of Brandon, our community suffers the same sadness our neighbors in Rutland face, on a lesser scale. We too have addiction problems that are tearing our families apart. We are a community of proud people who have lost many industrial jobs to the economy over the years. A community that struggles economically, that works hard to attract new businesses and residents to our town. Our community has invested in our police department to provide safety and security to its residents. We have also funded a new recreation department to engage our citizens young and old alike to offer opportunity and activities that engage all who live and visit here. Our Chamber of Commerce works diligently to reflect the needs of our community while looking for new prospective businesses to enrich our town. As hard as we all work to improve on what we have to offer, there continues to be the underlying deterioration of the fabric we are constantly trying to improve upon.

As the Chief of Police in this great community, I struggle with the same problems most law enforcement officers in Vermont face. Budgeting, personnel retention, and funding opportunities to assist us in our mission of providing a safe healthy community, while trying to assist those with substance abuse problems by directing them towards a more productive and healthy life through treatment. As you know from your visit to Rutland County, a new methadone clinic has recently opened, and as helpful as it may be, it can barely address the needs of those who need its services. As a Chief of Police with limited resources it is imperative that I partner with members of the Vermont Drug Task Force and other federal partners such as the DEA and ATF. Our federal prosecutors offices have done an outstanding job of prosecuting those who traffic in illegal drug activity and profit from the downfall of our neighborhoods. We are thankful to all of these partners for their support.

Community, Commitment, Integrity

While we are not ashamed to ask for assistance from others, we are continually reminded that not just our community, but many others in Vermont are asking for the same assistance. Funding for the Vermont Drug Task Force has been reduced over the years to the point that investigators within the task force are stretched to their limits working to assist all of the agencies requesting their help. Without their assistance, I am unable to combat the sales of illegal drugs such as cocaine and heroin in my community as a result of a lack of personnel and the financial resources needed to protect the members of my community from the influx of these illegal drugs. I respectfully ask all members of the Judiciary Committee to think about their own neighborhoods and communities. I am certain that you all care deeply, and want what would best serve your own communities. I ask only that you hear our calls for assistance, and understand that while we all will continue to work collaboratively to address the issues we face here in Vermont, a key component of the solution lies with law enforcement. Without the necessary means to investigate and prosecute those who infect our communities by trafficking illegal drugs, we are simply treading water. We need whatever resources can be made available to help us retain our way of life that we cherish, and will work diligently to utilize those resources with evidence based solutions.

Honorable members of the Senate Judiciary Committee, I thank you personally for the opportunity to provide testimony and to Senator Leahy personally for his leadership and his true connection to Vermonters.

Thank you,

Christopher Brickell
Chief of Police

Community, Commitment, Integrity

James M. Candon Jr.
Jericho, Vermont 05465

20 March 2014

Dear Senator Leahy and members of the Senate Judiciary Committee:

I retired from the Vermont State Police as a Captain nearly 16 years ago. I have been alarmed by the epidemic of drug addiction in Vermont and wish to get my views to you for consideration. One of my career assignments was as a prescription drug diversion investigator from 1981 – 84.

There can be little doubt that a fundamental cause of the opiate epidemic has been the abuse of LEGAL PRESCRIPTION DRUGS. There has not, however, been a conversation about how these prescription drugs became available for such widespread abuse. Nor has there been a conversation concerning what is going to be done to stop these drugs from being widely diverted for abuse in the future. The conversation appears to have jumped over the abuse of prescription drugs to the topic of heroin and putting a stop to heroin distribution. I am not suggesting that heroin interdiction is not important because it is. It was mentioned at your hearing that there were 21 heroin overdose deaths last year in Vermont. It wasn't mentioned that last year there were 48 overdose deaths due to prescription drugs, most of which were opiates! (See Vermont Health Department Report at http://www.documentcloud.org/documents/1061492-od-fatality-report-3.html)

In the many public discussions, including your hearing in Rutland on Monday, there was no one present that spoke with authority on the diversion of Rx drugs. Nor was there barely a mention of what real steps, other than the Vermont Prescription Monitoring System, were being taken to prevent future Rx drug diversion and abuse. Is there any doubt that the abuse of prescription opiates such as Percodan, Percocet, OxyContin, Fentanyl, Dilaludid, Vicodan, Codeine and other Rx painkillers have been a huge part of the opiate addiction epidemic? And is there any doubt that these drugs are prescribed and dispensed by doctors and pharmacists in our state? Are we naïve enough to think that these drugs aren't being diverted from our local pharmacies, doctors, hospitals, nursing homes and clinics but are all brought in by drug dealers from Massachusetts and New York?

For a variety of reasons, no serious emphasis has been placed on preventing the abuse and misuse of LEGAL prescription drugs in Vermont in the past 20 years or so. As a matter of fact, political pressure has been applied to further limit the inspection of records in pharmacies by diversion investigators due to privacy concerns and HIPAA. The pressure has come from pharmacists, privacy advocates and the ACLU. Another reason is a lack of interest by law enforcement. In Vermont forever the overwhelming focus has been on ILLEGAL drugs by law enforcement and prosecutors.

Diversion enforcement is not simply responding to complaints of forged prescriptions and conducting criminal investigations. Diversion enforcement goes way beyond that. The duty is to safeguard access to prescription drugs of abuse (controlled drugs) and to provide assurance that these drugs are being properly used for legitimate medical uses according to the rules, regulations and law. This is accomplished by conducting regular compliance inspections of records kept or maintained in accordance with the laws and regulations for the prescribing, dispensing and administering of these drugs. These rules apply to not only pharmacies but hospitals, clinics, nursing homes and doctor's offices where drugs are kept and distributed.

There is a popular notion in Vermont that we are going to solve our addiction problem with treatment. . The theme that "drug addiction is a chronic disease like diabetes and high blood pressure" is very popular currently. The hope is the new Vermont Prescription Monitoring System and the new MAT (medication assisted treatments; methadone and buprenorphine therapies) will make significant progress in dealing with the current epidemic. I'm hopeful as well. With these new strategies come unexpected problems. For example, the diversion of buprenorphine is all ready a significant problem. The VPMS will identify new cases of doctor shopping. Vermont needs strategies to prevent the abuse of controlled prescription drugs. Affective diversion enforcement is one! Actually the need for diversion enforcement will increase. I have found no plan to deal with uncovering diversion in the health care profession. Those that work in a medical environment where controlled drugs are widely available are vulnerable to abusing prescription drugs and it is not uncommon. Those that are licensed to order drugs from wholesalers like doctors and pharmacists are particularly vulnerable. It is an occupational hazard similar to working with money in a bank. Without outside inspections, bad things will happen.

Drug diversion efforts in Vermont suffer due to these fundamentals:

1. Failure by Vermont policy makers to understand the public health and safety damage that can occur when there is a lack of over site to the distribution of dangerous (controlled drugs) which are legal and prescribed by doctors and dispensed by pharmacists and others in the medical field.

2. Failure by policy makers to recognize the insidious attraction that prescription drugs have regardless of ones standing in life. This is particularly dangerous for those that work with these drugs in the health care professions. Drug addiction by doctors, pharmacists and nurses is not an uncommon occurrence.

3. There has been an insufficient level of attention given to prescription drug fraud and abuse by law enforcement and those assigned the specific "duty" to enforce the laws and regulations concerning the prescribing, dispensing and administering of controlled prescription drugs. This includes the states attorneys and the Attorney General. (See applicable Vermont statutes at: http://www.leg.state.vt.us/statutes/sections.cfm?Title=18&Chapter=084)

4. There is a prevailing view by policy makers in Vermont that prescription records in a pharmacy are "private medical records" and therefore should not be open to inspection by law enforcement without a search warrant. This sentiment needs to change in regard to dangerous controlled drugs in schedule II – V. Why is it that the State of Vermont inspects restaurants, elevators, vehicles, scales, beauty parlors, and even income regularly without search warrant requirements? Yet there is strong resistance to inspecting prescriptions of controlled drugs in a pharmacy even when these drugs have caused such tremendous addictions and loss of life. The state policy makers should stand up forcefully to this resistance

much like the Vermont Supreme Court did in State v Welch in 1992.
http://libraries.vermont.gov/sites/libraries/files/supct/160/op90-392.txt

5. The federal Health Insurance Portability and Accountability Act (HIPAA) has
   been used by the ACLU and others in Vermont to block diversion investigators
   access to prescription records without a search warrant in Vermont pharmacies.
   To see a full report on this topic see the Vermont Department of Health report to
   the legislature entitled Vermont 2006 at
   http://healthvermont.gov/admin/legislature/documents/Act205_med_privacy.pdf)

Legal prescription drugs are much preferred by drug abusers either to recreate or to
support a habit. They are commercially produced, powerful and safe especially when
compared to heroin. When a drug abuser can get them with a prescription from a doctor
they are very inexpensive. The schemes and scams utilized by determined drug abusers to
get prescriptions for these drugs are fabulously inventive and clever. Why do doctors
prescribe to these drug abusers? There are a variety of reasons and none of them good.
Elderly doctors, drug addicted doctors, naïve doctors and deceitful doctors are the targets
of drug abusers. The resale street value of these drugs is phenomenal.

A doctor can only prescribe controlled drugs for "legitimate medical purposes" and are
disallowed from prescribing for purposes of drug detox or maintenance.
(http://www.deadiversion.usdoj.gov/21cfr/cfr/1306/1306_04.htm). A pharmacist under
the same law has an equal and corresponding responsibility with the doctor to dispense
the drug only for a legitimate medical purpose. A properly trained and experienced
diversion investigator reviewing records of a pharmacy, including controlled Rx files, can
easily spot patterns that are inconsistent with legitimate medical purposes.

21 CFR part 1300 (http://www.deadiversion.usdoj.gov/21cfr/cfr/index.html) sets out in
detail the rules regarding controlled Rx drugs. When a medical professional is registered
with DEA either to prescribe or dispense controlled drugs, they are required to know and
follow the regulations. The regulations define all the essential rules that must be
followed.

Thirty three years ago as a young detective, I started a one man diversion section in the
drug unit at the Vermont State Police. I was given this assignment because of my
previous experience investigating pharmacies for the Medicaid Provider Fraud Unit at the
Attorney General's office. While conducting the Medicaid investigations I learned much
about the prescribing, dispensing and record keeping required in the distribution of these
drugs.. For the next 2-3 years as a diversion investigator, I conducted inspections in
pharmacies throughout Vermont. I no longer have my records but I would guess that I
inspected 50 pharmacies throughout the state. Vermont law gives diversion investigators
access to order forms, stocks of drugs, and prescriptions for controlled drugs in the
pharmacies. (Controlled drugs are drugs that are subject to abuse. They account for
approximately 10% of the drugs dispensed by a pharmacy. The controlled drugs
prescriptions in a pharmacy are kept separate and apart from the other 90% so that they
are easily accessible for inspection. So, inspectors DO NOT have unfettered access to all
prescription files – just the 10 %). In the course of my work I was able to identify and
arrest several drug abusers for doctor shopping, forging and altering prescriptions and
other scams. But what was shocking to me and for which I had not been fully prepared
were the cases showing doctors and pharmacists and nurses involved in diverting drugs.

In one case an elderly country doctor was selling written Tussionex (a schedule III narcotic) prescriptions for $10 each. Drug addicts from across the state flocked to this doctor for these prescriptions before he was shut down and retired by the Board of Medical Practice. In another case, a cancer doctor was stealing Demerol (a schedule II narcotic) from his patients and shooting himself up on house visits. When another detective and I met him in his office we asked him to roll up his sleeves. He had injection wounds up and down both arms. Criminal prosecution of him was declined by the prosecutor and he was sent off to rehab and thereafter supervised by the Board of Medical Practice. In another case, I visited a pharmacy in southern Vermont after finding a lead in an ARCOS report (http://www.deadiversion.usdoj.gov/arcos/#background). At the pharmacy I inspected the DEA 222 order forms and observed that the pharmacist had ordered several bottles of Deodorized Tincture of Opium (a schedule II narcotic). I then noted that he had only a small amount of DTO on hand in the store. I then reviewed his schedule II prescription file and noted there were no prescriptions for DTO. I confronted him with these facts and asked him what had happened to all the DTO? He then admitted he had a "business man's stomach and was self medicating for it" This case was prosecuted and the pharmacist pled guilty to Unlawfully Dispensing in court. In another case I arrested a doctor's wife for forging numerous Dexedrine (a schedule II stimulant) prescriptions in her husband's name.

Inspections of the pharmacy's records sometimes uncovered shortcomings that were not criminal in nature but that were out of compliance with the rules nonetheless. In these cases a report outlining the shortcoming would be submitted to the appropriate licensing board for whatever action they wanted to take.

In the early 1980's Vermont had a prescription drug addiction problem. Most of it was hidden and had gone unnoticed for a long time. I was asked by superiors to put on a training class for all the detectives in the Vermont State Police. I did this by traveling the state and making presentations. Eventually all detectives had received familiarization level training on prescription fraud and abuse. Before long I was promoted and transferred to another assignment. I did have the opportunity to train my replacement for a good period of time. His name is Bill O'Leary and he did a fine job.

Looking back on my career, being a diversion investigator was the most satisfying assignment of all. The reason is - not only was I solving crime but I was getting those folks that were drug addicted a chance to regain their lives. For most addicts, standing in front of a judge in court was hitting rock bottom. Their recovery could begin at that point. Those that were not criminally prosecuted were referred to the professional licensing boards and had the opportunity to begin recovery.

I am very disappointed that Vermont has suffered the terrible epidemic in recent years. I particularly feel for the families of addicts who actually suffer the most. Now the taxpayers need to fund millions and millions of dollars in drug treatment. Much of this problem was avoidable! Having an aggressive drug diversion unit that proactively did their job would have given early warning and prevented much of it from happening at all. I fear that policy makers still don't understand how much can be accomplished with a proactive diversion enforcement program. I'm fearful that policy makers lack the courage of leadership and the political will to demand a first rate diversion unit with access to the necessary records.

In closing I would like to make the following recommendations to the Committee:

1. Please include in your hearings some testimony from experts in Rx drug diversion. All states have diversion units and there are very knowledgeable folks available.

2. Be careful who you listen to in law enforcement regarding the drug epidemic. I noticed the list of witnesses who testified on Monday in Rutland included no one who had a background in diversion. Diversion work is very different from illegal drug enforcement. In diversion work there is no glory and cops are not attracted to it. I compare a diversion investigator to an IRS agent. You require no undercover cars or attire, you don't need to work with sophisticated electronic equipment, you don't get to make undercover drug buys and you don't get to kick doors in. You spend your days looking over records. It is very unglamorous work and very different from undercover drug work. It requires a unique set of skills, knowledge and experience. And it is tremendously rewarding.

3. Clarify HIPAA so that diversion investigators can perform the necessary inspections having access to records of controlled drugs without the need for a search warrant. HIPAA has really hampered law enforcement in Vermont as indicated in the Health Department 2006 report mentioned earlier. (http://healthvermont.gov/admin/legislature/documents/Act205_med_privacy.pdf)

4. Please provide some political leadership in emphasizing the need for effective diversion units in the states to combat the scourge of drug addiction by legal Rx drugs. The arrangement has always been that DEA Compliance would handle enforcement at the manufacturing and wholesale distribution level while the states would be responsible for enforcement at the retail level in the individual states.

Thank you for considering my comments.

James M. Candon
Captain, Vermont State Police (retired)

Dear Senator Patrick Leahy

I am writing on behalf of the 5-Town Drug & Safety Alliance – Treatment Committee. The 5 towns referenced are Bristol, Lincoln, Starksboro, Monkton, and New Haven – all in Addison County, Vermont.

The 5-Town Drug & Safety Alliance was formed in 2012 in response to multiple break-ins of cars and homes, thefts, burglaries, and drug related crimes in the 5-Town area. Out of a Community Forum three committees were formed: Prevention/Education, Law Enforcement, and Treatment.

The Treatment Committee is a coalition of concerned citizens, community and religious leaders, and members of the counseling and medical community.

We laud Governor Shumlin's State-of-the-State speech about drug addiction. Bravo! The points made highly resonated with the views of our committee. We strongly believe that we cannot arrest our way out of the problem. Because of the high level of demand for opiates, an arrested dealer is soon replaced by another. There are huge profits to be made.

Recovering the lives of people suffering from the disease of addiction requires three important ingredients:

1) Medication Assisted Treatment (with drugs such as Suboxone/Buprenorphine)

2) Intense Counseling

3) Long term Peer Based Recovery (like Narcotics Anonymous)

The committee has worked diligently to advocate for Medication Assisted Treatment, Counseling, and long term Peer Based Recovery for addicts. The Counseling Service of Addison County and private Licensed Drug and Alcohol

Counselors are providing excellent support for addicts. So, too, is the Turningpoint Center in Middlebury with its peer based recovery programs.

The lack of Medication Assisted Treatment in Addison County is a huge problem. Addison County has only 1 MD providing Medication Assisted Treatment whose practice has only recently started, and who treats at most 15 addicts at the present time. This is an important, but tiny step forward. Just in Addison County, there are far more addicts in need of recover that are not being treated.

To our knowledge, Addison County is the only county in Vermont with only 1 MD providing treatment. The Counseling Service of Addison County (CSAC) and Porter Hospital have worked on this problem for a number of years. Because of the lack of MDs providing Medication Assisted Treatment, they are proposing a Medication Assisted Treatment Clinic for Addison County, which is under consideration for funding by the Vermont Health Dept.

This drug problem is about lives. It is about the lives of residents who have had property stolen, cars broken into, and more. And most definitely, it is about recovering the lives of addicts so they can be freed of the disease they suffer and be happy, productive members of our communities.

We hope that you can help in our effort to fund a Medication Assisted Treatment Center in Addison County, and other counties in similar positions.

Thank you very much.

Bb Donnis, on behalf of:

5-Town Drug & Safety Alliance – Treatment Committee

Letter Published by the Addison Independent Newspaper on 2/6/14

To the Editor of the Addison Independent

We applaud your front page article "Police tackle drugs in Bristol" (1/27/14). Chief Gibbs and his team have done an outstanding job over the past 3 years in apprehending dealers and thieves. Bravo!

As members of the 5-Town Drug and Safety Alliance – Treatment Committee we would like to add to what Chief Gibbs has said. He said "...we're not foolish enough to think (dealers) won't be back." A big motivator for dealers is profit: "a bag of heroin that sells for $5 in Boston can sell for as much as $30 in Bristol."

We would add that not only is there profit, there is also demand. There is a huge demand for heroin and other drugs in Bristol, the 5-Town area, Addison County, and all of Vermont. To quote Governor Shumlin in his State of the State speech: "The crisis I am talking about is the rising tide of drug addiction and drug-related crime spreading across Vermont". Demand creates supply.

In addition to police efforts to arrest dealers and thieves, we must find ways to reduce the demand. This means that Prevention (education), and Treatment must be equally pursued with Law Enforcement. Again, from Governor Shumlin's speech: "Chief Justice Reiber and so many others who are in the thick of this struggle have concluded, we must bolster our current approach to addiction with more common sense. We must address it as a public health crisis, providing treatment and support, rather than simply doling out punishment, claiming victory, and moving on to our next conviction."

There are various effective treatment approaches to help get people off drugs and into recovery. They include Medication Assisted Treatment, Outpatient and Residential Counseling, and Peer Based Recovery Programs such as Narcotics Anonymous and other services at the Middlebury Turningpoint Center. Treatment includes all of these. Are they always successful? No. Are there relapses? Yes.

However, a significant percent of addicts treated stay clean for the rest of their lives.

We are talking about lives here. Certainly we are talking about the lives of theft victims, but, we are also talking about recovering the lives of addicted individuals and their suffering families. Are they bad people? No. They are people with a disease. Governor Shumlin:"...Dr. Holmes got it right when he noted that addiction is, at its core, a chronic disease. We must do for this disease what we do for cancer, diabetes, heart, and other chronic illness: first, aim for prevention, and then eradicate any disease that develops with aggressive treatment."

Do we have local treatment options for addicts in Addison County? Some, but not enough. We have highly trained Licensed Alcohol and Drug Counselors at the Counseling Service of Addison County and in private practice. We also have many Peer Based Recovery programs at the Turningpoint Center. However, there is currently only 1 doctor certified to provide Medication Assisted Treatment in AC. We need more doctors willing to treat addicts. Today, most AC opiate addicts must travel to Rutland or Burlington for treatment, sometimes multiple times per week. For addicts who have lost their car either to support their habit or for DUI, this presents a huge hurdle to obtaining treatment, and is often a showstopper for addicts to seek treatment. We need more Treatment options right here in Addison County.

What can we do as residents of Addison County? We can advocate for treatment in Addison County doctors' offices and/or a clinic. Ask your doctor to seriously consider providing treatment. Sign a petition of support (available from: 5TTreatment@gmail.com). If you know someone in your extended family or circle of friends who is addicted, encourage them to seek Treatment. They can start by calling the Counseling Service of Addison County (388-6751). They can also call 2-1-1 for referrals for treatment.

As Governor Shumlin stated: "...the time has come for us to stop quietly averting our eyes from the growing heroin addiction in our front yards, while we fear and fight treatment facilities in our back yards."

Solving the "Drug problem" is more than just arresting dealers and thieves. It also requires prevention of addiction through education, and multiple treatment options (including Medication Assisted Treatment, counseling, and peer based recovery programs). It is about recovering the lives of people who have the disease called addiction.

Thank you!

Bob Donnis for:

The 5-Town Drug and Safety Alliance – Treatment Committee

A coalition of concerned citizens, community and religious leaders, and members of the counseling and medical community.

Thank you for the opportunity to weigh in on this critical public health issue. As addiction treatment clinicians at the Brattleboro Retreat, our perspective on the opioid addiction epidemic in Vermont (and beyond) comes from the front lines. In the past ten years we have witnessed a dramatic increase in the number of people seeking treatment for opioid dependence, which includes addiction to both opioid prescription analgesics such as oxycodone and street drugs such as heroin.

The disease of addiction affects people of all ages and from all walks of life. However, in our experience, the current opioid addiction epidemic disproportionately affects young people. The costs of this problem to individuals, families, and communities have been nothing short of devastating. We absolutely believe that effective approaches to this problem will require intense, collaborative efforts that must include treatment professionals, prevention specialists, schools, families, and state, federal, and local government agencies.

Efforts aimed at reducing the supply of opioids should include additional efforts to help prescribers become even more cautious when they prescribe opioid analgesics. The Retreat has already contributed to physician education on savvy prescribing and we are aware of other efforts across the state. That said, continued education and greater interaction with primary and specialty care providers regarding the appropriate use of opioids for both time limited and chronic pain is essential. This includes greater awareness of how to safely manage chronic pain in general, as well as specifically in patients who already have, or at high risk for, the disease of addiction.

We know that timely, effective addiction treatment ultimately supports prevention efforts. Children of parents in recovery from addiction will be less likely to become addicted themselves.

Because people with active addiction are ambivalent about seeking treatment and following through, we support the increased diversion of addicted individuals from incarceration to treatment. Treatment is both less expensive and more effective.

Lastly, increasing public education efforts on the causes and effects of opioid addiction will help reduce demand (prevention), and make treatment options for those who are already in trouble more appealing.

Yours sincerely,

Geoff Kane MD, MPH

Chief of Addiction Services

Brattleboro Retreat

Kurt White LICSW, LADC, CGP

Director of Ambulatory Services

Brattleboro Retreat

Many years ago, in the process of creating RAMP (Rutland Area Mentor Program), I visited families living in the NW neighborhoods and other similarly blighted areas of Rutland. I remember the shock I felt at seeing the conditions under which people lived in the city I called "home." Talking with mothers and children in smoke-filled rooms, I heard despair and longing. I saw holes in the unfinished sheetrock, stained ceiling tiles, doors hanging by one hinge, and the ashtrays spilling over onto rusting TV tray tables. I saw crowded sleeping spaces, panes of broken window glass, and the hollowed-out faces of poverty.

Two summers ago, I volunteered on the Pine Ridge Lakota Reservation in South Dakota. The housing looked a lot like the homes I visited in Rutland many years ago. The voice of poverty sounds the same. It looks the same; skin color does not change the despair and longing.

When RAMP was created, I was a teacher at the Rutland Area Vocational-Technical Center known as "voc." Some of our students grew up in those smoke-filled rooms and came to us from a legacy of perceived culpability for their poverty; a reinforced awareness that the "voc" was all they should aspire to in life. Often bullied in school and at home, they breathed the air of drug abuse and they learned to adapt themselves to the behavior they saw as "normal." Becoming the "them" that nobody wants to be was their trajectory.

When I read Larry Bayle's comment in the Herald coverage of the recent judiciary hearing, I thought, "He's hit the nail on the head."

How *do* you fight classism? A week or so ago, I spoke with a twenty-three year old young man who talked about how he has always felt that Rutland is "different." Having grown up here in a relatively affluent family, he keenly felt the differences between people and felt diminished by classism. He used the term, "classes." He was not talking about school. Some of his ideas are worth hearing and talking about. As they say on TED talks: ideas worth spreading.

Rutlanders refer to "upper" Baxter Street and "upper" Grove Street, and "down in the Gut." A kind of "us and them" culture has emerged over the years. I believe it is that ethos which is as the core of the current problems plaguing Rutland, not the least of which is grinding poverty.

If there was ever a time for change, it is now. The energy feels different this time around. I have witnessed more than a few "resurrections" in Rutland and this one *is* different. It feels like it has a future. Driven by so many residents who are committed to making change happen, there is every chance for success.

My concern is that we give voice to *all* the people. We need to give voice to the 25% of people living in poverty who are concentrated in the NW neighborhoods and elsewhere in Rutland. We need to be careful that we do not condemn people to the story that has been created around them. We need to hear what they know and have learned. We do *not* need to tell them what we have learned *about* them without their consultation.

In the service of better understanding the "drug problem" the question we must be asking now is not only why people take drugs, but *why do people stop.*

We know, from the volumes of research, that poverty and social isolation go hand in hand. We know that family, employment, and status within the community are factors that counterbalance drug use and abuse/addiction. It is harder for people with nothing to say no to drugs. We must be mindful that their perception of *nothing* is not necessarily ours. We must be slow in reframing the drug problem and be careful not to reinforce a culture of "us and them."

As a working RN, I am aware of the public health ramifications of substance abuse and its effects on our children. In changing the trajectory of our young people in this community, we need to take the long view. In the near term, we need to create a healthful environment that runs into the future and hears all the voices that make up this splendid place called Rutland.

In closing, I see blue sky and the long shadows of the end of another day spreading across the golfcourse and I am glad to live in Rutland. And I am lucky to have a window on such beauty.

Respectfully submitted,

Regina M Kohlhepp MS BS RN-BC

Dear Senator Leahy and Judiciary Committee Members:

Let me start with the life story someone has shared with me: Born to parents who were first generation high school graduates born in the Depression, grandchild of immigrants who fled poverty and hopelessness, his parents worked their way up to homeownership. His mother developed a serious mental illness when he was 9 and his siblings were 7, 6 and 3. His father and grandmothers filled in the gaps when his mother was unable. He grew up with fear, lack of trust and frequent embarrassment. He describes himself as one of the lucky ones, since he learned and grew from these formative experiences and developed the strengths that his loved ones and supporters exhibited, and few of the weaknesses. He survived rebellious teenage years that might have wound someone with less support in jail, DCF custody, or worse. He was given the support and encouragement to go to college then graduated into an earlier recession and took the scarcity of good jobs as an excuse to go to post-graduate school which in those days could be had with summer-job earnings. He wonders just how much support and opportunity it took to deflect him from a fate much like many of those struggling in Rutland right now.

I am a long time Public Defender and Prisoners' Rights Attorney working in Rutland for the last 27 years, and prior to that in Jersey City, New Jersey, so I am intimately familiar with the individuals whose addiction and/or poverty (and lack of the "grace of God" that kept my acquaintance, and so many of us, from such a fate) often blights once healthy communities. I speak also as the mother of three Rutland High School graduates who are proud of their school and their community, the most recent a 2010 graduate (he's best friends with Carly Ferro's brother). I am the Vice President of the Rutland County Parent Child Center Board of Directors, and a member of Project Vision. I was one of the committee members who helped design and implement Rutland Drug Court Grant and sat on its Oversight Committee (until the funding ran out for one hour a week!), and for nearly 27 years, I have been involved with numerous other community and school programs and events.

Thank you for bringing the Judiciary Committee to Rutland as we once again bring the community to the struggle. The Rutland Drug Court received Senator Leahy's support in applying for the grant that funded its design and three year implementation. As part of that broad state and local effort, we learned of the need to design a program that would attract the folks who would best benefit from it, and we received training about best practices in understanding and treating the medical condition of addiction, the young people whose brains are still developing, and addicts with a "brain on drugs", particularly one on opiates.

Besides the Drug Court, earlier community-wide efforts resulted in the Wits End parent-of-addicts information and support group, the Turning Point Club, The Boys and Girls Club, and many other great and necessary services to help addicts and their families find treatment and support for them and their families.

As a result of the community wide involvement and the training we received,

Rutland's State's Attorney has continued to support the Drug Court and most recently announced that he will support Rutland in following Chittenden County's lead by implementing a Rapid Intervention program here. This means that addicts accused of crimes committed to support their addiction can now agree to seek immediate treatment for their disease and avoid criminal prosecution if they follow the imposed requirements successfully. This is a crucial tool to meeting addicts when they are most willing to go to treatment, and will hopefully result in convincing them that recovery is a better path than addiction, and adding them as a strength rather than a detriment to the community. Since a court case may take months to resolve, the early start when they are most willing adds to community safety as well. Ideally, this will be part of a seamless system from Diversion, to Early Intervention, to Drug Court. I believe it requires another system wide effort by the criminal justice partners. Using early assessments (containing confidential information), agreed to by addicts while high, to publicly make determinations about treatment need and success will not attract most users. This is a good idea that needs further discussion and precautions to be successful.

The federal drug court grant Rutland received a decade ago also taught those involved in its creation about the Teen Brain and the brain on drugs. Treatment, and family and community development require a recognition that young brains are different. Every parent knows the experience of a child becoming moody, irrational, lacking foresight, self-centered, rude, feeling invincible, and selfish. Science is now learning that this is because the brain does not complete development until the mid-20s, so the young brain is not yet capable of thinking about the effects of their behavior on other people; they lack insight. Add alcohol or other drugs and a young person's brain, which is wired to form new connections, becomes deeply habit-forming. A drug like heroin actually destroys areas of the brain that give us the capacity to love and empathize. This can result in cognitive deficits that cannot be re-wired without long hard work. Opiates artificially activate brain centers and turn off the body's ability to make its own. This means the brain suppresses its natural reward centers, so that the only thing that brings happiness is taking the drug again. This brain chemistry explains why addicts often relapse after six months of clean time. The brain needs to practice how to deal with risky situations. Users need to learn to develop social and emotional relationship skills that the brain stopped learning at the time the drug use began. The best programs have the right kind of support that users need at this time. Sanctions in Drug Court, on Probation or elsewhere can't be based on our frustration with the participant's progress, but must be based on what works best for this individual.

A well operated, informed system provides rewards and sanctions, carrots and sticks. And the awareness that manipulative and other skills an addict needs to survive remain for some time. There can be progress and then regression. It takes strong, knowledgeable and compassionate treatment providers and other professionals to not write them off as sociopaths. These folks in the throes of addiction are not necessarily likeable. It is easy to view them as "the other". But there's nothing better than seeing who that person really is, as the shroud of addiction diminishes, and the healing of the brain begins to take hold. Surprisingly often, you hear their mom or dad say, the daughter that I know is back! Joy comes from the number of folks in Drug Court who thank judges and prosecutors for supporting them into solid recovery. Some say they have never had the sustained support of a caring adult before.

Crucial to the success of treatment systems is the education of the community to recognize that recovery is NOT about will power and strength of character. Blame has no place here.

One shortcoming of Rutland's earlier start on addressing the heroin and attendant crime problem was the fact that the recognized need for a methadone clinic fell to political pressure. The opening of the West Ridge Center for Addiction Recovery in Rutland last year fills the gaps created by the use of buprenorphine which does not ease all cravings, can be redirected to misuse, requires many more trained doctors than the community has, and does not have the necessary wrap around social services that medication assisted treatment requires to enable those in recovery to succeed. Those who had made their way to daily 3 hour trips to a methadone clinic had difficulty finding work hours to fit with that schedule, missed segments of their family's life, and spent countless scarce family funds to pay for the travel. Hopefully this new focus will also help ensure that medical, including dental, professional become aware and well trained about the dangers of prescription pain medications.

The struggling communities in Rutland are not filled solely with addicts but also people who grew up with the generational effects of poverty, or abuse and neglect. Nearly all drops outs had parents who did, nearly all men who strike a woman grew up abused or saw their father abuse their mother. Many, many of the child sexual abusers are themselves victims of their caregiver's abuse when they were the age of their victims, leaving them stuck at that immature age without appropriate treatment. It is not all about power and control. Much is about breaking a cycle of poverty, abuse and hopelessness. This is not a simple or short term process. Programming needs to be informed about trauma, addiction, the brain and poverty. The generational lack of resources my friend was fortunate have sufficient support and resilience against underlies most of school failure, domestic violence, child sexual assaults and susceptibility to escapes like drug use. As Governor Shumlin said, "none of us should be content until all Vermonters, including those who are born into poverty, have the same opportunities to succeed and flourish as the most fortunate. Our best prevention against drug addiction is to create jobs and opportunity for all Vermonters. By providing the best early childhood education in America. Every Vermonter regardless of income, has the chance at success – living, working, and raising their family right here in Vermont."

Rutland is fortunate to have community leaders that bring together a community-wide focus on issues such as poverty, addiction and the crime needed to maintain addiction. I would like to share some of the short and long term lessons and questions that I have taken from the successes and occasional shortcomings of these efforts. The predominant issue, naturally, is the lack of sustained financial and community support for the outcomes of community efforts. This means that great programs like Wits End can't pay for the essential therapeutic support person of late, that small programs suffer by living week to week, no one is overseeing the community-wide gaps and duplication of programs.

What are the other challenges now? We have not yet been able to begin to address the rampant "us against them" mentality that is wide-spread in our community and nationally. Thankfully, Project Vision is hard at work on community building. Both reality and the spin of the national "news" fight us on this at every turn. The poor don't trust "us". Why should they? They believe that politicians say what they have to to be elected, and what they read and hear is either black or white, depending on the source. How does anyone know what the truth is, or who you can trust?

This national break down is at least n part caused by the growing gap between rich and poor. The remnants of the upper middle class and the rich strive to escape the realities of modern life post-Great Recession by building more gated communities, making their purchases on line and otherwise avoiding any contact with the poor, leaving the poorest to their own islands of poverty, where those who fled leave those islands so undiversified and unsupported that they are left to rot. The anger is bubbling just below the surface of those who feel left behind in this economy, working several jobs to make ends meet, and hearing gross generalizations about the poor and minorities being the root cause of unaffordable taxes and other evils. The Great Recession is still upon us.

So, how to get Rutland (and elsewhere) to see that THEY are WE! I was shocked when a conservative friend who recently retired to an essentially gated community down south asked the 4 liberal democrats we were travelling with whether we had noticed a big increase in the number of homeless people. Maybe you can run but you can't hide. Bandaids won't do it. We've seen what happens when we try to divide and conquer, which we have seen prominently in the "Stand your Ground" laws and their aftermath. After the remarkable testimony from the Director of the Burlington Boys and Girls Club, the Rutland Herald reported a frank comment from one of the employees of the Rutland Boys and Girls Club. How do you address the class divide? Like the Rutland County Parent Child Center, these small organizations, making a small dent in turning around the future. However, the kids who attend these programs tend to be viewed as, and in fact largely are, the poor. And many of the poor are generationally poor, parents and grandparents raised in a time when we understood even less about how to grow a healthy community. How did the voters deny the Rutland County Parent-Child Center's request for $13,500. on Town Meeting Day? How could they disagree with Rutland's need to help support their great work with families and young children with comprehensive, high-quality, family centered services designed to enable their success in and contribution to the community. Our "Learning Together" program works with young parents to provide counseling, academics, parenting, job readiness, interpersonal skills, coaching to help prevent child abuse and neglect, reduce dependency on public support, give parents increased competence, improve health outcomes for parents and their babies, avoid family violence, improve life skills and lessen or prevent repeat pregnancy. Our "Strengthening Families" program reduces risk and promotes protection of children by offering support for families who are dealing with stressors that may not otherwise meet criteria for "at-risk" services, developing positive relationships with parents to make them more comfortable seeking support, especially those who may be reluctant to disclose concerns or identify behaviors or circumstances that may place their families "at risk" and helping families build and draw on strong and healthy support networks w/in their families and the community.

And who are the so-called "They" anyway? One or two straws more or less and it would have been my friend, maybe any one of us. While it is no doubt impolitic to say, many of the young adults who are accused of selling drugs here are from elsewhere. What we are learning, however, is that they are mere cogs in a larger machinery, part of a disposable and unlimited supply of young men at risk in their own communities coming here in the hopes of bettering their lives. Jailing them is incredibly expensive, and they are immediately replaced with other low level dealers from elsewhere. Or they are from here, selling just enough to get their own needs met with the profit. We incarcerate more people than nearly any other nation. It costs $50,000 dollars or more per year to do so. By doing this we separate intact families, and add to family instability as well as raise our taxes. We are dooming the next generation already.

At criminal court we see the mothers and other support systems of the young out of state kids arrested for drug dealing, who have found someone with a car and the money for the gas and have driven 5 hours, and arrive stunned at the allegations against a kid who was doing well until... Their kids striving, just like ours, but in a community devastated by poverty, drugs and crime the choice as they see it is hop the train and sell these drugs and bring the money back, or live a life of hopelessness. Yes, some escape; a testament to the human spirit. But some come here, ply their wares, maybe even impregnate a local girl who feels similarly hopeless, or is addicted and takes him in for the drugs and some money. These are our community's kids and issues, too. We can't incarcerate our way out of that problem either. As Gov. Shumlin reported, nearly 80% of those incarcerated are either addicted or in prison because of their addiction. Add the folks with untreated mental illness, and those with learning disabilities and you reach nearly 100%, I suspect. And we know the cost of this is unsustainable, and destructive to families and communities.

Rutland Police Chief Baker and Project Vision Chair Joe Kraus have told you much about Project Vision's great work in building and utilizing strong connections and relationships within the community to begin to address the issues and restore a sense of community to Rutland's struggling neighborhoods, and I won't repeat that information here. Crucial is the emphasis on citizenship and community which West Ridge has said is "a key component of a successful recovery program".

Also at issue is that many of these kids and their families are involved in many social service agency programs. Project Vision is rightfully proud to be eroding the silos that work with different family members, different family issues, and yet the challenge will be how not to end up turning this into a gossip and retribution outcome but strong, positive community redevelopment. We need to agree on the results we seek and set out plans based on those outcomes. Another challenge will be to reduce the lack of trust in police, government, courts, and the do-gooders. For example, Chief Baker's willingness to say that we can't arrest our way out of this situation, that police need to work with service providers to achieve healthy outcomes, must be balanced by the need to protect family confidences and privacy. Confidentiality of private information is protected for a fundamentally important reason. We believe that people can grow and change and should not be defined by educational deficits, mental illness, youthful indiscretions. The challenge is how we can ensure that this work with the whole person and the whole family is successful not only when things are going smoothly, but also when they aren't. Knowing that addiction is a chronic, relapsing disease, only adds to the complexity.

What unique struggles do we have? There are persistent gaps in services. Public transportation is weak. How can you get a kid with no family resources to soccer tryouts and practices, to the Boys and Girls Club? We have to ensure that family members who touch many caring (or burned out) support systems receive coordinated, not redundant support. We have to teach our support systems how to view the problems in a way that lessens burnout, and to address it when it inevitably occurs.

I have a bias against grants as funding mechanisms. Implemented solutions must be fully realized and permanently sustained. Many a young and smart recent grad has been hired to run a local program only to leave when the grant runs out, replaced by someone who lets the group's energy lapse, or sometimes just never sets a next meeting. This happened with the well- yet poorly-named Heroin Committee, and other regional early success stories. A good leader is well worth keeping and nurturing! That takes long term financial support that short term grants don't offer.

The Great Recession still holds us in its grip. Homes are under water or in foreclosure, out of state banks with no regard for the vitality of the community abandon buildings, and those former homes then attract crime. The federal HAMP law is thwarted in its best practices by out-of-state banks that have acquired other banks and have such confusion in their records that the court process becomes yet another process of frustration and expense to the already strapped homeowner. In Rutland we see the effects in the derelict and abandoned properties in the neighborhoods which police say attract drug dealers and buyers, further depleting a neighborhood's resources. Might Congress help us unclog the legal machinery to refinance or reclaim these properties and return them to a valuable asset in our community? Some Vermont towns voted recently in favor of the creation of a state bank which would create a "10 Percent for Vermont" program in which 10 percent of Vermont's unrestricted revenues would be deposited in the State bank, with power to leverage this money to fund some of the unfunded capital needs and to create loans which would help create economic opportunities for Vermonters. We could put people to work and repair our failing infrastructure at the same time!

As a result of these concerns, through Project Vision we have reached out to the local landlord group whose monthly newsletter is read by 400 Rutland landlords, to try and elicit their involvement in working on the blight that is holding communities back.

The neighborhood in which Project Vision has its first focus currently has 21 vacant or blighted buildings, which severely affect the quality of life in the neighborhood. The hope is to restore, or demolish and replace with attractive energy-efficient homes approximately half of those structures in the next four years. Vision partners are approaching smaller funding sources to underwrite spruce-up projects, encourage gardens, creating more open green space and public art projects, and considering the feasibility of converting the vacant former assisted living facility into a community asset. Many bright spots have already appeared. The Dream Center on West Street, created through the personal commitment of Linda Justin and her husband Bill, now mentors neighborhood boys and girls, and helps families in need. What was once called Bums' Alley, the major pedestrian access to shopping, services, and transit from northwest, which had been a site of heavy drug activity, is now a revitalized bike and pedestrian access, the Baxter Street Alley. By Spring, in conjunction with the Vermont Farmers' Food Center (also known as the Winter Farmers' Market, situated on a prominent once-blighted property, now home to a bustling indoor winter farmers market), Baxter Street Alley will become another blooming bright spot in the neighborhood.

Rutland is blessed with great attributes, and is an exceptional place to live and work. However, not only in Rutland, but throughout America, drug sales, addiction and related issues are holding communities back. Project Vision is working on some of the larger issues behind this trend by enlisting the community to work together to find new approaches and implement some that have worked elsewhere. We believe that by working together we can accomplish more than we ever could working alone. This is hard work, but we believe it will be successful. We will surely need support.

I appreciate the Judiciary Committee's visit to Rutland and the opportunity it has given me and so many others to discuss our concerns and our ideas.

Respectfully,

Patricia M. Lancaster
Mendon, Vt.
March 21, 2014

The Honorable Senator Patrick Leahy
United State Senate
Washington, DC 20510
March 21, 2013

Dear Senator Leahy:

Vermont is battling an unlikely giant in opioid addiction, and the action being undertaken at the local, state, and federal levels show promise in helping to find solutions to this vast public health epidemic. Here in Vermont, we have benefited from the Senate Judiciary Committee's Focus of finding "Community Solutions To Breaking The Cycle Of Heroin And Opioid Addiction" with your field meetings throughout the state, and our own state initiatives to address the issue, highlighted by Governor Shumlin's directives laid out during his State of the State address this year.

I am writing today to call your attention to the efforts that are providing measurable positive outcomes in Bennington County regarding this problem that have been working specifically to reduce access to prescription medications due to the work of the **Bennington County Prescription Task Force**, a small working group that you may not have been introduced to by name or deed.

On Thursday, March 13, 2008, the Bennington Police Department, the National Association of Drug Diversion Investigators Inc. (NADDI), and the Southern Vermont College hosted a one day training seminar on prescription drug abuse and diversion, drawing a large crowd from the law enforcement, medical, and social services groups from the southern Vermont area. Peter Grasso from NADDI presented information on Pharmaceutical Diversion and included tips on how to proceed and what to be aware of within this issue as well as the topic of internet drug sales. Steven Kennedy from the Office of Professional Regulation (VT Secretary of State), Phil Ciotti (VT Department of Health (DOH), Board of Medical Practice), and Virginia Merriman (Medicaid Fraud and Residential Abuse Unit (VT Office of Attorney General) all presented about the vast problem with drug diversion in Vermont.

This wonderful forum proved to be the impetus to form a more focused and multidisciplinary group to address these very same issues in our region. The goal of our group from the outset has been to bring in a variety of people and organizations to one table for monthly meetings in order to address the problems that we all were seeing develop in the area and also throughout the nation. The center piece is reducing access to prescription drugs in the community and also providing education to our neighbors about the dangers of legal and illegal drugs. All of these enterprises have catapulted Bennington County to the top of the state's list when the DEA conducts their biannual drug take-back events (in April and October), despite our being the third smallest county in the state.

Positive gains have been realized by calling together members of: law enforcement (local police and sheriff offices), medical (doctors, administrators, and pharmacists), other government agencies (local and state, in the healthcare and judicial arenas), schools, the local health department, prevention teams, the recovery community, and other partners. We have successfully integrated efforts across these sectors in both the Northshires and Southshires, instituting a year-round program for taking back unused, unwanted, or expired medications throughout the county with three permanent collection sites. Not only are the police departments in Manchester and Bennington available daily for this intervention, but we have developed an efficient method for mailing medications to the Bennington Sherriff's Department. In fact, the Sherriff is available to send a deputy to an individual's house for pickup if that is more convenient. Additionally, the Bennington Police Department has recently teamed up with students at Mount Anthony Union High School and Career Development Center and fabricated a distinctive (and rather good looking) container for people to walk into the PD and dispose of their medications. This was a great partnership that combined the talent and ingenuity of the youth of the community, allowing them to witness firsthand the difference they can make in this fight.

The inroads with the medical component has allowed for peer-to-peer discussion and distribution of information about drug misuse. Our local hospital now includes information about proper drug disposal, and the physicians in the emergency room have changed their standards of practice to look at reducing the amount of medication dispensed through the emergency room. I have visited all of the Bennington area pharmacies on multiple occasions, championing the promotion of DEA take-back days and also providing education on the use of the DOH's Vermont Prescription Drug Monitoring System, which allows for the review of recent narcotic/controlled substances filled in the state to help determine if a patient is appropriately using these potent, addictive, and potentially dangerous medications.

All of these efforts were recognized at the Prescription Drug Misuse Prevention Strategies Learning Community Day, which occurred in Montpelier November 13, 2012. The Vermont Department of Health, cosponsored by the Vermont Criminal Justice Training Council (VCJTC), hosted a resource event in direct response to the Vermont Prescription Drug Abuse Workgroup Recommendations Report, outlining strategies in 4 key areas: Education, Monitoring, Disposal, and Law Enforcement. The learning community examined risk and protective factors and related evidence-based practices for prevention. Community teams had the opportunity for cross-regional sharing of the approaches currently being implementing in each of the key areas, with the following objectives:
• Increase understanding of basic information about the incidence, prevalence, and consequences of prescription drug misuse in Vermont
• Increase knowledge of the work going on at the federal and state levels addressing prescription drug misuse.
• Increase knowledge of actions being employed by communities around the state to address prescription drug misuse.
• Review and examine evidence-based approaches in addressing prescription drug misuse in communities.
• Learn how you can participate in efforts in your community.
It was an honor for our group to share what we are doing in Bennington County with members from across the state, including the Commissioner of the Vermont Department of Health, Dr. Harry Chen, and other members of the state's policy makers and law enforcement. This format allowed for networking opportunities and a glimpse into what other localities in the state were doing to address the objectives noted above, deepening the knowledge base for all in attendance and providing discussion points to be brought home to the local level.

Our group is proud of the difference we are making in the state and are now introducing new efforts to reach the families of every elementary, middle and high school students in Bennington County. We have designed two flyers stressing the importance of proper drug disposal via the options we have developed through the hard work of the task force, with graphics that are specific to either the younger or older child. Relationships have been formed at each institution, allowing for articles that have been written by the Bennington County Prescription Drug Task Force to appear in the school newsletters. Past topics have included the proper methods available to dispose of medications, the importance of family meals, and the influence of music and pop culture related to the use of drugs. These newsletters provide the parent with information about what their kids are being exposed to when away from the home, and a springboard to open lines of communication to help children to thrive in an often chaotic world around them.

The Bennington County Prescription Task Force has been meeting regularly for over five years and helping to shape our county's approach to the issue of drug misuse and abuse from a diverse section of community with the end goal of helping to reduce the financial and emotional burden that these problems present to our individuals, families, and communities. We are confident that the dedication of the team members have helped to implement favorable and sustainable changes that can be used as a model for the rest of the state and beyond.

Sincerely,

Michael S. Leake, BS Pharm, R.Ph.
Community Pharmacist
Bennington County Prescription Task Force
Bennington, VT 05201

I know it's the last minute but please, please consider our needs in Addison County.

1. A urine testing site like Burlington Labs - affordable-convenient
2. Intensive out-patient center - not a 12 step program but a real day program of treatment
3. Suboxone or methadone dispensary

I ask for these things because, if you or someone you love has gone through a residential program, you need follow up to succeed. You need and actually want to be held accountable by random urine screening. It helps to know that you'll never know when. If you have to drive to Burlington or Rutland, you may never get there because of work or travel restrictions. Meeting with a counselor for an hour a week is not enough to maintain a drug free life. You need intense outpatient therapy. Some people need drug replacement. Is it just a crutch? Yes, it's a crutch or tool to help get off opiates. If you broke your leg you'd use a cast and crutches. This is really no different. It's an aid to help healing.

Please find the means to provide our struggling addicts with real help.

Sincerely,

Mary Martin
Cornwall

Greetings,

March 25,1999 we received the knock on our door that no parent wants, a police officer came to notify us that a young girl had been left at the emergency room at Rutland Hospital, had died from a possible drug overdose and he had reason to believe it was our daughter Sarah. "...Would we come to identify the body?" My wife and I were devastated and numb to what followed the next few days with notification to our family and funeral arrangements for our beautiful, sweet and very intelligent nineteen-year old daughter.

Our family didn't fit the common perception of a "drug family". It did represent the profile of a much more mainstream family with teachers, social workers, healthcare (several nurses),clerks, building trades, an architect, law enforcement at the local and state level, and several also served the community and state as elected officials; one was even a former lieutenant governor. It was obvious that "common perception" was not accurate and how we perceived and addressed the problem of drug addiction needed to change.

We went back to work and tried to continue our routines as a rural mail carrier (Pat) a florist (Kathy) and as parents to Sarah's two younger sisters ages seventeen and eleven. But life would never be the same. We felt lost and alone with so many questions and so few answers. Were there signs that we missed? What could we have done? Who could we turn to for answers and support? Where do people go for help with problems of addiction? Why do people use drugs? Why did our daughter have to die? How do we survive as a couple and as a family? When will this nightmare end?

Over the next year or so we tried to find answers by attending every twelve-step program and support group and by meeting with the local services. There was no place that totally filled our needs as parents of an addict; we were at our wits end. We decided to start a group on our own for education and support for families of addiction. My wife, Kathy, said "That's it! We'll call it Wits End because that is where we are." We drew up a plan and brought it to the newly formed Rutland County Heroin Committee, a collaboration of the Rutland City police, Rutland County Sheriff Department, Rutland County Courts system, Vermont Health dept, Rutland Mental Health, and now Wits End was there to represent the parent perspective. A commitment was made to work together to do what we could to solve some of the problems drugs had brought to our community. (This was in response to the kidnapping and murder of Theresa King by several young men who were high on drugs.) We (the Rutland County Heroin Committee) met for several months and some very positive outcomes were realized. The drug court was instituted, Turning Point recovery center was opened and with initial support from the ADAP (alcohol and drug abuse program) of the Vermont Department of Health, Wits End Parent Support Group found a meeting place at the Spectrum facility for teens at risk which was in Rutland at that time. This was in 2001.

In the years since forming our group we have steadily grown in numbers of families attending and in the scope of problems addressed. As parents and not trained professionals, Kathy and I have learned much about addictions but we have always had a licensed counselor present for their expertise for the questions that arise that we are not qualified to answer. We strive to educate families about addiction, the signs and symptoms of drug use ,the appropriate responses to take, strategies for "raising the bottom "in a safer and quicker manner, the treatment services available and the glossary of treatment, what has worked for others and what doesn't work, and we support the family in whatever path they chose to follow.

Now in 2014 the Drug Court program is a proven success and is spreading to other areas of the state, the Turning Point centers for addicts in recovery are in most counties of the state, and the Rutland Wits End model has been duplicated in many other locations, too, (although sometimes under another name.)

We strongly believe that greater inclusion of parents in this "War on Drugs" is not only mandatory but is also fiscally responsible. Parents have the strongest and most consistent influence on our youth. Parents have the most passion for positive outcomes for their children no matter what age they are. Parents don't have to be hired or vetted or voted into office. They are "ex-officio". What we need to help in this war is support of the proven programs such as Wits End to continue and expand the education and support of parents and families of addiction.

Thank you for all you do for this state and country,

Kathy and Patrick Martin
Co-founders, Wits End

U.S. Senate Judiciary Committee,

First of all, I would like to thank Senator Leahy for his Help and Concern in Rutland Vermont, Vermont, and all States in the U.S.A. We all have a Drug Problem and need help in combating it.

I'm not from Vermont, but have lived here since 02/02/1979. We have owned our home in Vermont since 1991 on Park Avenue. We have seen Problems come and go on this street over the years. But nothing Like This. I have seen Rutland and the State of Vermont go from being a place to raise a family to not a good place at all. Most of all here in Rutland.

At this time of my life I feel that Rutland is not a city that I would want to raise my family in. I feel that I can say this as I have spent a life time working with kids here.1977 to now. I have been a Coach, in football, baseball, basketball, an umpire for 24 years, ran the score clock for Rutland High and Jr High. Spent 10 years as a Substitute Teacher. The one thing that I can say is that I have given my all to the city of Rutland Vermont.

Now, I try to teach my grandson and others right from wrong if they ask or need help. I'm a small part of this city and will not give UP ON HER. I along with other fathers stopped problems on my street once before and WE WILL helps do it once more.

Once more thank you for coming to Rutland and SEEING our story First Hand. It meant a lot to this City of ours.

SEMPER -- FI

Michael F. Moran
Rutland, Vermont

US Senate Judiciary Committee   March 21, 2014
Senator Patrick Leahy, Chairman

I attended the "Community Solutions to Breaking the Cycle of Heroin and Opiate Addiction" hearing held in Rutland VT on March 17, 2014. My name is Kristi Morris and I am a resident of Springfield VT, which is located approximately forty miles southeast of Rutland. We too are plagued with the presence of opiate and heroin activity in our community, as is many other Cities and Towns within our State.

I must commend the US Senate and particularly Senator Leahy and Representative Welch for hosting and attending the recent hearing. In order to combat the growing drug epidemic, local, state and federal efforts must partner together if we are to ever curb the activity surrounding the use of illegal drugs. It has become painfully obvious that we must further our efforts to educate, treat and rehabilitate our citizens and young people with regards to drug use and its devastating effects.

Springfield is much smaller than Rutland having a population of approximately 9200 residents. Our community is situated on the VT – NH border along the Connecticut River and has Interstate 91 passing through our eastern township. This makes commuting from the Springfield MA area a mere one hour and forty five minutes. The State of New Jersey is also within a travel time of six hours, plus or minus.

I mention that community and those two States because they are the areas of supply for the product that is introduced into the southern part of Vermont, and particularly, our Town. The I-91 corridor makes it easy for those traveling to Vermont for illegal drug distribution to those willing to become involved with the illicit substances.

The Town of Springfield has a stagnant grand list, since the demise of the much heralded machine tool industry that we enjoyed post WWII. Since the last company left Springfield in the 1990's, we have struggled to revitalize our community but have made great strides in attempting to diversify our job market and local industry.

Because of the paralyzed grand list, our residents are burdened with the highest property tax rate in our State. Our community is a full service Town having Police, Fire, Highway, Water/Wastewater, Library and Parks and Recreation departments. We also are burdened with the second highest road mileage for a Vermont community.

Our residents have supported our educational system by voting to bond for consolidating and rebuilding of our elementary schools. Our aging infrastructure has required that we additionally bond for rebuilding our wastewater treatment facility, dilapidated water system and storm water separation.

Springfield has recognized that we must have sound educational and infrastructure systems if we are to grow our community and attempt to provide for a sound economic development opportunity. However, the stagnant grand list means that the tax burden sits squarely on the shoulders and wallets of our taxpayers.

We have partnered with the State of Vermont in many areas. We have a correctional facility, State Department of Motor Vehicles, Public Safety Division of Fire Safety, DCF, etc. to name a few State agencies, and many, many other groups and organizations.

We also have Springfield Hospital, the regions health care facility operated by the federally qualified Springfield Hospital Medical Care Systems. They are a much needed resource in our Town and they own and operate the Hospital, Edgar May Recreational Center and the local clinic, which operates out of one of the previously vacant machine tool buildings.

All these services coupled with the Springfield Health & Rehabilitation Center and several elderly housing units place an enormous requirement on our tax base for providing the necessary services and demand that our infrastructure be maintained.

I recognized that Springfield is not alone in our great State for the criminal activities associated with problems centered on illegal drugs. Rutland is not alone with regards to the violence and crime surrounding drugs and many other cities and towns have similar problems.

In July of 2012 we had one epiphany on our downtown streets that has forced us to look at areas of concern and address those that have brought the drugs into Town. Two of our residents inadvertently met on Main Street followed by a fight and subsequent discharge of a hand gun. This immediately provided an eye opening, made for TV, situation that played out in our community for our citizens to see and hear right on our main street.

I was, and still am, a member of our Town's Select board and I vowed to work on understanding the problems associated with the drug activity and associated criminal activities. Moreover, in the past two years, I have attended many seminars, forums and community discussions on finding possible solutions and uniting the various agencies.

The Vermont League of Cities and Towns (VLCT) have several meetings in a calendar year. I have attended their local Government Day and Town Fair Day and talked with our State legislators regarding the illegal drug activities. Chief Baker, of Rutland, sponsored community forums in his City, which I have attended to understand how he is coordinating efforts to combat their community's drug problems.

I have attended Vermont's Court Administrators Tri-Branch Task Force meetings and several other forums including the Public Safety Commissioner, Court Administrator, Department of Corrections Commissioner and Director of Probation and Parole. My purpose for attending is to understanding how Vermont's system works with regards to the criminal activity and what actually happens when arrests, arraignment s are prosecutions are made.

What I have learned is we have several gaps in how criminal activity is processed and handled. In Vermont, a person can be arrested for an illegal activity, arraigned in court and released on conditions. This enables them to be back out on the street in a minimum amount of time, without serving any incarceration. The obvious conclusion here is that they often return to the same activity that brought them there in the first place. Secondly, when an incarcerated person is paroled, or served their maximum sentence, the agency that is to follow up with them is severely under staffed.

The most glaring gap, that I have realized, is we have an enormous need or requirement, for treatment and rehabilitation services for the growing drug population. Though many agencies and services exist for their treatment, they too are extremely lacking in staff to expeditiously treat and process the users.

Springfield is working toward providing resources to counter some of these activities and have looked at the Rutland model for guidance and opportunities. In our next budget cycle, we have added an additional police officer but we recognize that we cannot arrest our way out of the problem. Our correctional facilities are at capacity and the cost to incarcerate is enormous compared to treating them on the outside.

We recently passed an ordinance requiring our landlords to register their buildings to identify the apartment locations with regards for firefighter safety and protection. We have also enacted another ordinance associated with dilapidated buildings. These are similar to what Rutland and other communities have done or are doing to "clean up" the housing stock and commercial building appearances.

Springfield is fortunate to have an active police presence and services. Because of the high tax rate of our community, we appear to be under staffed when compared to communities of similar size and population. For this reason, the State has been very cooperative in partnering resources and providing additional aid through their Drug Task Force unit. They conducted a sweep in the summer of 2013, which netted over thirty participants in illegal drug activity.

The State Senate has introduced bill S295 this legislative session, which is geared toward processing those arrested for drug use. The bill is designed to provide the necessary services for treatment and rehabilitation for those arrested as an alternative to incarceration. I applaud the efforts of this bill and look forward to the House adopting it this year.

Vermont's judiciary is also addressing those who travel from outside of the State to sell drugs by adjusting or increasing penalties for those with intent to distribute opposed to the casual user. Crossing State lines with high volumes of drugs, particularly opiates and heroin is looked at with more severe penalties.

Senator Leahy's and the Judiciary Committee's recent effort in Rutland are commendable and, as stated previously, I applaud the efforts to communicate from the federal legislative level.

Springfield is a desperate Town looking for solutions against the drug activity, not just in our community but for the State as a whole. It is encouraging to see the recent local, regional and State efforts to combat the problem. I am further encouraged to see that the federal government, particularly the Senate Judiciary Committee also has an interest and is looking at the problem.

We could stand with our hand out asking for money for more police officers, more jails, more judges and prosecutors but that is not the perceived solution. It is widely recognized that we cannot arrest ourselves out of this epidemic problem. Further, it is recognized that we cannot incarcerate all those involved with drug activities.

What has become obvious is the need for additional educational support for our young people and the need for treatment and rehabilitation services. The only successful way to reduce the opiate and heroin drug use is to remove the users. There will always be a market with criminals waiting to make a sale. You arrest and prosecute one and another is waiting to step into his place. The more we can reduce the addicts and users, the less enticing it will be for those traveling into our region and state to sell their products.

Springfield has many local and State agencies to deal with treatment and rehabilitation. However, we do not have a methadone or health care clinic specifically to treat drug addiction. If users or addicts cannot find or get treatment, their option is to remain a user and the cycle continues. It is imperative to break this cycle and enable the users who want to find help or need the counseling intervention to have access to treatment.

Finally, as stated previously, I believe it is imperative that the local, state and federal governments need to partner together for solutions. No one community is exempt from the affects of heroin and only a cooperative effort can and will be successful. Rutland, Springfield and other cities and towns cannot do it by ourselves.

Vermont is a rural State with a small population but with a big problem. It is my vision that our proud State can work together with local and federal government, be proactive give us back our pride and educate, treat and rehabilitate our families, neighbors, friends and citizens who are affected and devastated by drugs.

I would like to thank the Senate Judiciary Committee for their time in recognizing the problem, their efforts and consideration for action and solutions on behalf of all Vermonters and those in the New England region.

Mr. Kristi C. Morris
Town of Springfield resident
Member Springfield Selectboard

Summary:

- Increased educational efforts
- Increased treatment & rehabilitation agencies
- Increased penalties for Inter-State trafficking
- Increased Inter-agency cooperation.

My son Michael had a knee injury almost ten years ago, he was 21 years old. He was living in the North East Kingdom. At the time, I was not overly concerned since he reported that he was going to physical therapy and was given medication for the pain. He was prescribed OxyContin. I had not heard of the medication but was happy that he was doing well and would make a full recovery. Michael was prescribed OxyContin for 6 months.

After Michael's recovery from his knee, he moved to Addison County. Michael worked construction full time, getting married and buying a home. During these years, I was so proud of him. He seemed happy, hiking, camping and snow shoeing and playing his guitar during his free time. His wife divorced him after 8 months. He continued to work but was showing signs of depression. I had asked him to see a counselor to help him get over his depression or maybe he needed an antidepressant. He said he was doing okay but was having a hard time making it financially since he was now responsible for his house and truck payment. I suggested getting roommates to help out with the bills until he made a decision on what to do with his house. In the time frame of approximately a year, I and my husband helped Michael financially. He always seemed broke even though he was working and had roommates living with him supposedly helping him with bills. Michael also lost weight. He went from weighing 210 pounds down to 145 pounds, he was skin and bones. I had made appointments for him at the open door clinic here is Addison county because I thought he must have some illness or cancer. Michael continued to work and said he was fine. He would come to family functions and be half asleep in the chair, not playing basketball with his cousin or visiting with other family members. At this time I still had no idea of what was going on. At the end of the year, Labor Day week-end, Michael and his girlfriend at the time, went for the week-end to visit his sister in Saint Johnsbury. His sister called me on that Saturday and told me Michael was taking drugs. She searched his knapsack while he was sleeping and found pills, then used pill identifier to find out it was Suboxone. Why was he taking Suboxone? She said he was addicted to pain medication. I called Michael and told him he needed to meet me on Sunday, alone when he got back from seeing his sister. He met my husband (his step father) and me on Sunday afternoon and we asked him to tell us what is going on? He said that he had been taking pain medication and was addicted to it. He said that he had tried to stop but couldn't. He also said that he had been using heroin because it was cheaper than buying OxyContin on the streets and he was buying Suboxone to try and get off heroin. In his words, "Nobody wants to be a heroin addict." He agreed to go into treatment and that's when the process took longer than I would have ever thought. He called tow treatment centers each afternoon after work with me (I wanted to make sure he was making the calls) He had to tell his history of drug abuse which started with the OxyContin for his knee ten years ago.

He talked of his use of using oxytocin recreational occasionally. He told them of his heroin use and attempts to quit. He was on a waiting list that could be 6 months long. He was supposed to call daily and they would note that he was still on the waiting list to get in. In the meantime I was extremely emotional. As a parent, questioning why did I not see the signs? I spent hours on the computer educating myself self on heroin and opiate addiction, signs and treatment. On September 19th, Michael moved away to his sister's, away from all of his connections for drugs in Addison County, leaving his roommates at his house (they too were heroin and opiate users). We tried to get them out since they were not paying rent and did not have a lease. The police would not kick them out, what a mess, but that is another whole story.

Michael went through withdrawal at his sister home and she was able to get him into the BART program. This meant that he was treated with a prescription of Suboxone and had random drug tests to make sure that he was not taking other drugs. He did very well with the program and was back to work in Middlebury and had plans to keep his home. He also came back with a new girlfriend who had a past of drug abuse but had been clean for two years (at least that is what she claimed). Michael would drive up to the BART program once every two weeks for his prescription and random drug test.

After a year and a half he was discharged from that program because his girlfriend stole his prescription and he started buying prescriptions on the street again. A relapse and, with the information that I have read, it is not unusual for this to happen. He again moved to the Northeast Kingdom to get away from drugs and start over. He found a job and was working 65 hours a week; remember 15 hours is at time and a half and buying drugs off the street.

This lasted from March 2013 until October 2013. As of October he is clean at least he has said he is. He sees a psychiatrist once a week to treat his depression and addictive behavior. This is a long uphill battle for my son and our family. Since finding out about Michael's addiction to opiates and heroin, we have learned that many of our friends and neighbors have experienced drug issues in their families with their adult children.

I don't have a solution but something has to change. I think that doctors have to be more aware of what they are prescribing for pain medication, especially to a young adult. I strongly believe that teens need to be educated on the seriousness of even taking medications on a recreational use. Opiates are much more addictive and can lead to heroin if not treated. I really do agree with my son that once a person is addicted to opiates that they want to stop but can't without some sort of treatment, maybe a combination of Suboxone and therapy. It is common knowledge that there is a crack house here in Addison County, I am sure the police are aware of it, but what good would it do to arrest these people if there is not a place to put them. I am sure that these users want help too. I really believe that having treatment available when people seek help is important. I don't know how long the wait list is for treatment but as I said earlier, it was a six month wait to get in 4 years ago. When Michael was in the BART program he was able to work full time and contribute to society and I think that is important component of the recovery process.

Thank you for listening.

Donna Quesnel

Hello,

My son is presently in the St. Johnsbury Correctional Facility, once again for drug use, and was sent there through his P.O. His constant returns to jail have been because of relapsing. Although I don't blame his P.O., because she has to do what she has to do, there must be something else we can do to keep my son alive. He, as well as so very many others, are incarcerated for the same thing. What I am pleading to you is that if these people are in jail for these issues, why can't we get a good program, like the Discovery Program, which has been closed, a mandatory requirement for these people? It seems it would be the best time to get to them, when they are clean from drugs and vulnerable!

Nobody what this is like unless you've been through it with your own son or daughter. Dan is going to be 33 next month. He has a beautiful soul, but a terrible addiction that does not want to release its claws from him. Although I am terribly exhausted and frustrated, I am not going to give up on guiding him and so many others like him for help.

Thank You,

Alberta Randall

Senator Patrick Leahy
US Senate Judiciary Committee
opiod_hearing@judiciary-dem.senate.gov

Re: Hearing on "Community Solutions to Breaking the Cycle of Heroin and Opioid Addiction"

Dear Sen. Leahy & Committee Members:

To begin, I thank you both personally and professionally for taking the time to address this vital concern to our community, state and nation. We have certainly seen the effects that drug addiction has had on our community and know that it is going to take a lot of effort to reverse the disturbing trend we've seen over the past several years. Even in rural Addison County we have seen increases in crime including drug trafficking, theft and breaking and entering in secluded neighborhoods where residents have not had to even keep their doors locked in the past. Our local and state police have done a tremendous job investigating these crimes and have made many arrests resulting from these investigations getting criminals and drugs off our streets. Of course, law enforcement is only one piece of the puzzle that needs to be in place to sufficiently address the concerns of addiction and we will never "arrest our way out of this problem".

Boys & Girls Club of Greater Vergennes has been a leader in Addison County's community prevention efforts over the past decade. The Club is a local, community based organization that has served youth and families of our community since the summer of 1999 with after school recreation and youth development programs and activities.

The Club has played an active role in alcohol, tobacco and other drug prevention in Vergennes and Addison County since 2004 when the organization partnered with ANWSU to apply for (and received) Vermont Department of Health's (VDH) New Directions Grant. Implementation of this program supported student led prevention efforts in all ANWSU schools and the Club's offering of evidence based prevention programming to elementary and middle school students during the school day. This grant also allowed Vergennes to make a strong presence in the Addison County prevention community, with staff from the Club regularly attending county wide meetings and activities.

In 2007, the Club continued its prevention efforts with the award of a Strategic Prevention Framework (SPF) grant from VDH. This award was intended to make a "population based" impact on underage drinking and high risk drinking in our community. The Club was able to implement a variety of projects during the three year grant program that involved youth in prevention efforts, informed parents and adult community members of the dangers of underage drinking, increased DUI enforcement efforts and raised public awareness of the risks of underage drinking and high risk drinking. Overall, however, perhaps the best outcome of the project was the way it brought different aspects of the community together to focus on these issues. A lasting, collaborative approach to prevention, treatment and enforcement of drug and alcohol issues is vital to making any real change in the community.

The Club's Prevention efforts have continued with VDH funding for a Combined Community Prevention Program from 2011 to the present that has enhanced drug and alcohol prevention programming by adding financial support for tobacco control and obesity prevention projects. This combined effort has allowed us to address all of these issues from a public health perspective that can focus on population level efforts to affect changes in community norms as well as individual and family based efforts to promote healthy behaviors and discourage harmful choices.

We firmly believe that to effectively address the cycle of heroin and opioid addiction we will have to engage in a broad based, community wide effort to attack the problem from all angles – enforcement, prevention and treatment. Strong efforts have been made in all of these areas in our community.

Local law enforcement has reached out to local residents to gather information, has utilized staff and cooperated with other departments to conduct investigations and have sent a clear message through arrests made that drug activity is not welcomed in our community. Unfortunately for every individual taken off the street it seems there is another one ready to move into their place. A continued and consistent enforcement response will be necessary to continue to address the issues.

Access to treatment for addiction seems to have improved over the past year or two. Where we used to hear of lists of more than 700 people waiting for treatment services, it is my understanding that these waiting lists have come way down. Although Vermont's "hub & spoke" model of accessing treatment, especially medically assisted treatment services, has helped many addicted individuals there are still many that struggle to gain access. There are still few doctors in Addison County willing to serve as "spokes" prescribing medication and managing treatment for those addicted and the physicians that are able to provide this service can only serve a handful of cases while still maintaining their practice and supporting other patients. Travel to "hubs" is also a challenge for addicted individuals. Public transportation in Vermont is limited and for those that cannot afford private transportation an hour long drive to a clinic is daunting at best, especially with the regularity required for medically assisted addiction treatment.

Prevention is the key to reducing demand for the drug in the first place and simply cannot be ignored in addressing the issue. In our community we see two distinct levels of prevention as well – secondary prevention to provide support and encouragement for those in recovery, and primary prevention to provide education so individuals never start down the path of opioid addiction. We are fortunate to have a wonderful recovery center in Addison County that has been able to implement several programs to provide support for those in recovery including peer support and "recovery coaches".

We have undergone many efforts aimed at primary prevention of opioid addiction in Addison County including support for "Drug Take Back Days", community educational forums, and showings of the film "Hungry Hearts" that highlights opioid addiction in Vermont. We believe these educational and prevention efforts are vital to keeping addiction in the forefront of people's minds and to help the general public understand that heroin addiction can very well start with that bottle of pills in the medicine cabinet prescribed by your doctor for pain relief.

We also believe that there is a deeper issue at hand that has not received the same attention as heroin and opioid addiction over the past few months. As a youth serving organization, our first concern is always how our actions, both positive and negative, have an effect on children and what our efforts look like from a child's eyes. With this in mind, there are few things as damaging to our prevention efforts as the way society deals with alcohol and marijuana.

Thanks in large part to societal norms around drinking, we see many more young people using alcohol than any other substance in Vermont. Unfortunately use of marijuana is not that far behind. According to the 2013 Youth Risk Behavior Survey, administered to middle and high school students every other year by the Vermont Department of Health, we see that alcohol and marijuana use among our young people far outweighs the use of heroin and prescription drugs.

Lifetime Substance Use Among VT High School Students in 2013			
	9th grade	12th grade	Total
Marijuana	23%	52%	39%
Alcohol	41%	74%	59%
Prescription Pain medication	8%	14%	11%
Heroin	2%	3%	2%

From our own research and experience, we know that in many cases this alcohol is provided by parents, older siblings and friends that are not aware of all the health risks associated with underage drinking. In the media young people are barraged with alcohol advertising and the ubiquitous glorification of drinking and drug use throughout popular culture – movies, television, music and of course, endless (virtually unpoliced) videos on YouTube and other internet outlets.

This onslaught has not been limited to the entertainment arena either, as it has expanded to news reports and government with two states legalizing marijuana and many states talking about following suit, including our own Governor who chose to use his State of the State address to raise awareness of addiction.

As a result of these factors, we see very accepting attitudes among Vermont's youth regarding substance use. Again, according to the 2013 Youth Risk Behavior Survey we see that more young people believe it is wrong to smoke cigarettes than marijuana and 2/3 of Vermont's high school seniors think that it is ok for them to drink alcohol.

Percent of students who think it's wrong for someone their age to...			
	9th grade	12th grade	Total
Smoking Cigarettes	85%	62%	75%
Drinking Alcohol	66%	34%	49%
Smoking Marijuana	71%	45%	57%

Thanks to well-funded prevention efforts under the Master Settlement Agreement with tobacco companies and a pubic shift in perception of tobacco we have seen a decrease in favorable attitudes around tobacco use and a decline in smoking among both youth and adults over the past ten years. Unfortunately the health concerns about alcohol consumption and marijuana use have not been given the same level of awareness and it shows, even among young people's perception of their parents' attitudes. In the same 2013 Youth Risk Behavior Survey, we see that while high school students still feel that their parents disapprove of substance use more than they do themselves, they still perceive more acceptance of alcohol and marijuana than tobacco.

Percent of students who think their parents disapprove of...			
	9th grade	12th grade	Total
Smoking Cigarettes	95%	85%	90%
Drinking Alcohol	84%	60%	74%
Smoking Marijuana	89%	76%	82%

While we would never suggest that we take our eye off the ball that is the opioid addiction issue, we believe there is a great disservice being done to our young people if we don't look at these "lower level" drugs as well. Many people will argue whether or not marijuana and alcohol are considered "gateway drugs" that lead to abuse of "harder" drugs, however, one cannot really argue that those that do try heroin and prescription medication usually start with alcohol and marijuana first.

We have grave concerns that the state and national climate regarding marijuana use and the increasing talk of legalizing the drug makes our prevention work even more challenging. We often hear "the war on drugs isn't working" or "prohibition didn't work with alcohol" as reasons to throw up our hands and regulate the legalization of marijuana. We believe that giving up is not the answer to the problem, but only the start to making our problem worse as it pertains to the health and safety concerns we have seen with opiate and heroin addiction.

We need to address all of these public health concerns the same way:

- Strong partnerships with enforcement, treatment and prevention agencies and organizations
- Well-funded efforts to support local and statewide efforts
- honest and open discussion about the problems we face related to substance use and abuse

We believe with a comprehensive effort we can and will have an impact on substance use and public health. Thank you again for your time and attention to this matter and I greatly appreciate the opportunity to contribute to the discussion.

Sincerely,

Mike Reiderer
Executive Director
Boys & Girls Club of Greater Vergennes
PO Box 356
Vergennes, VT 05491
(802) 877-6344
bgcvergennes@comcast.net

21 March 2014
Dear Sen. Leahy:

I am a transplanted Vermonter, having lived in many other areas of the country after growing up on a farm in upstate NY. I moved to the Northeast Kingdom when I got married twelve years ago. My husband is an adjunct professor at Lyndon State College and a paralegal in the Caledonia County State's Attorney's Office. I am the director of the Heart of Vermont Chamber of Commerce -- the chamber for the Hardwick area and surrounding towns. We are grandparents, we live and work in Vermont, pay Vermont taxes and have an interest in the viability of our state and the conditions and challenges under which we and our neighbors carry on our lives.

The drug problem in Vermont came to my attention shortly after I started meeting our neighbors and getting involved in our community. One day I walked into our post office and the lobby reeked of pot as did the gentleman who just left the building. The postal clerk, a longtime resident, apologized and then told me about who was dealing -- and what they were dealing -- on a local basis. When I asked her, "Why don't you tell the police?" she replied, "We have to live (here) in this town." She felt that the police weren't in a position to help.

Another person -- a long time business owner whose grandchildren had switched from public schooling to homeschooling -- told me that there had been heroin sales and drug deals taking place in the back of the public school buses.

Sometime later, while sitting in the newly opened Claire's Restaurant in Hardwick, I was looking out the front window to enjoy the sunset and watched a drug deal take place in full view of myself and rush hour traffic. The realization that there was a serious problem here was inescapable.

My viewpoint is that drug and alcohol abuse are a problem but they are also a symptom of underlying problems within Vermont. Drug and alcohol abuse are not going to go away until the causes of the underlying problems are handled. Specifically, people turn to these "solutions" when they no longer have hope, they are not producing (i.e. they cannot find employment), and due to ignorance of the effects of drugs and alcohol.

At the risk of stating the obvious, if drug use in Vermont is an "epidemic," *it is a epidemic which is fueled by both illegal drugs* (heroine, meth, etc.) *and also by the misuse of prescription drugs.* Cheap heroine makes its use much more prevalent. Over-prescription and "on demand" prescription of pain killers, anti-depressants and mood altering drugs such as Ritalin has made their consumption commonplace rather than rare. We have become a society that reaches for a pill rather than looking for real solutions to our problems. Our present approaches to solving addiction appear to prolong and exacerbate the problem.

One ex-addict told me, "Don't give more drugs when getting someone off drugs. Try non-traditional programs that do not involve handing out more opiates. Build a meth clinic and you'll have more drug users. What a great place for some to get free drugs amidst the people actually trying to quit. Support of loved ones, families and friends is vital, but not if any of them are users. It's a temptation to fall into the same old routine. Being surrounded with non-users helps."

Having former addicts help users to get clean seems like a good idea. They know what it's like. They've been there.

If we are going to set up a system for diversion, then we need a system that actually works. The current system and past methods appear not to be working since we have more drugs on the streets. It's time we clamped down on the over-prescription and mis-prescription of drugs that so often are a jumping off point for the cycle of addiction. It's also time we had effective and early education on what drugs are and their effects so that we prevent kids from starting in the first place, rather than having to try to "cure" them later on.

Sincerely,
Maria Roosevelt

Iboga, the plant that Ibogaine comes from, is considered sacred in Gabon and Cameroon, where it grows. In the West, it has gained a reputation for its ability to treat opioid and other substance abuse disorders.

It is not a maintenance drug like Suboxone or Methadone. Ideally, it is administered in a medical setting after proper screening. It provides a relatively painless detoxification over a period of 36 to 48 hours. It gives a person a fresh start, reducing cravings and giving insight into past choices. Part of the way it does that is through its psychoactive properties. Those are also why it's had a hard time getting approved for use in the United States. Vermont is well-poised to go around that obstacle, in the same way that we've been in the forefront on medical marijuana, under the aegis of the tenth amendment of the U.S. Constitution.

Treatment works best when it's the addict's choice. Let's give addicts another choice for treatment, one that doesn't just switch what drug they are taking, but gives them a chance to put all opioids behind them. I encourage this committee and the rest of the legislature to learn more about this form of treatment.

Sincerely,
Bonnie Scott
founder of the "Vermonters for Ibogaine Research" group on Facebook
URL: http://freevt.org/vt/

Hi, my name is Vito and I am a resident of Rutland, VT. I do wish to add my voice to others in finding a solution to the opioid addiction afflicting our state. My views may be just an opinion, but I believe that by finding the essence to this matter, we may be able to tackle this problem from its roots. Many may just repeat the same ideas like tougher laws, or more police patrol, or even the suggestion to legalize all stimulant substances.

The people who want to stop the use and addiction of drugs need to be more informed to identify the users, activities, health effects, and social falls. The drug users must be informed that they are watched by the community. People willing to help may convince users to seek treatment on time to avoid convictions, high legal costs and social exposure.

Sincerely, Yours

V.M.

Breaking the cycle of substance addiction

The task to stop this epidemic may be in several ways. Inform the public to identify the users by exposing signs of intoxication and personality changes. Encourage community participation to watch for signs of trafficking that may aid the enforcement of laws. Tips may be received by anyone observing and not necessarily by residents. Anyone arrested regardless of reason should be tested for drugs.

Treatment expenses must be paid by the inmate and recovery must be a condition for release. This is a program that can be accomplished by informing the public by means of mass communication. Present a campaign why body and mind stimulants are illegal, how stimulants destroy individuals, families and relationships, why it is a national concern affecting economy, health, and education. Finally show why voluntary treatment is a solution that remains confidential. The campaign to reduce DUI and tobacco use is a success, so by exposing the dangers of drug use must be a campaign too.

Vito Moro 3/20/14

Coming Out of the Darkness

Harry Chen, MD
Commissioner of Health

Vermont is finding its way out of the darkness of opioid addiction. With the opening of West Ridge Addiction Treatment & Recovery Center in November, we marked a milestone in Rutland County and for our state. We now recognize addiction as a chronic illness, like diabetes and heart disease, requiring a similar approach to prevention and treatment.

Just as people with diabetes need medication like insulin along with lifestyle interventions, so too do people with addictions need medications like methadone or buprenorphine and lifestyle interventions to ensure the best outcomes: better health, steady work and a social network of support. The opening of West Ridge is especially meaningful for me, as a longtime former Rutland County resident and physician, but the real credit goes to the medical and treatment community, law enforcement, business leaders and neighbors who pulled together to make it a reality.

Addiction is not someone else's problem – it's our problem. Along with just about every other parent of young adults, I know several of their classmates who were well-adjusted kids with caring parents whose lives were taken over by the horrors of opiate addiction. Thankfully, nearly all are now in recovery and doing well.

At a cost of millions of dollars yearly, addiction is a problem we can't afford to ignore. And we can't forget the other immeasurable costs of poor health, broken families, unsafe and unstable communities. Addiction touches each of us.

Among the most innocent victims are newborn babies of women addicted to opiates. These are not "addicted" infants, but they do require special treatment at birth that fortunately prevents long-term detrimental effects. The vast majority of addicted mothers giving birth in Vermont are in treatment. From a public health perspective, this is precisely where we want them to be. We take pride in a prematurity rate that is among the lowest in the nation as a marker of our willingness to commit to our collective future.

Addiction stems from bad decisions, just like any of us might make to overeat or not exercise. But it quickly moves from a bad decision to disease. The end result is a chronic medical condition with profound implications for the individual and society. We must take the public health approach and confront addiction on all fronts – no one really expects we can arrest our way out of the problem.

With the opening of West Ridge, and BAART Behavioral Health Services in the Northeast Kingdom on January 1, we are implementing the Care Alliance for Opioid Addiction – the partnership of treatment centers and clinicians around the state using a Hub & Spoke model to offer medication-assisted therapy to Vermonters in need.

The treatment centers, or Hubs, will serve patients with complex needs. Hubs offer comprehensive assessment and specialty treatment with methadone or buprenorphine, providing treatment much closer to home for many. Connected with the Hubs are the Spokes – Blueprint for Health and primary care practices that treat patients using buprenorphine. Patient care, at a Hub or a Spoke, is supervised by a physician and supported by a network of community-based services aimed at our goal: enabling patients to be successful in life, work and as family members. This system of care gives a health home for people addicted to opiates. The federal government shares our enthusiasm for this model, acknowledging its innovative nature with enhanced federal start-up funding.

Two recent national reports underscore that all three branches of state government are committed to finding solutions. A report from the Trust for America's Health commends Vermont's use of all 10 nationally recommended strategies to reduce prescription drug abuse and overdose. A National Safety Council report credits our state as one of only three to meet all of its standards on state leadership and action, prescription drug monitoring, responsible prescribing, and overdose education and prevention.

As we work to address the demand side of the equation, we can't underestimate the power of prevention. We see hope and progress in the 2013 Vermont Youth Risk Behavior Survey results that shows use of tobacco, alcohol and prescription drugs by Vermont youth declined significantly from 2011 – all priorities for our community-based prevention efforts. Investing early in the health of young people clearly yields the best return on investment.

I believe we are on the right path.

www.ingramcontent.com/pod-product-compliance
Lightning Source LLC
Chambersburg PA
CBHW080009210526
45170CB00015B/1959